Hot Flashes

Hot Flashes

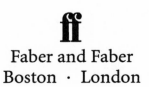

Women Writers on the Change of Life

edited by Lynne Taetzsch

ff

Faber and Faber

Boston · London

Introduction, Collection, and Notes copyright © 1995 by Lynne Taetzsch

The acknowledgments on pp. 177–179 constitute an extension of this copyright notice.

Library of Congress Cataloging-in-Publication Data

Hot flashes : women writers on the change of life / edited by Lynne Taetzsch.
    p.   cm.
  ISBN 0-571-19871-6 (hardcover)
    1. Menopause—Popular works. 2. Menopause—Miscellanea. 3. Menopause—
Social aspects. I. Taetzsch, Lynne.
RG186.H68   1995
618.1'75—dc20   95-21808
                                                                        CIP

Jacket design by Lorna Stovall
Jacket painting by Lynne Taetzsch

Printed in the United States of America

*To my sisters, Laura Kirsner and Mary Azerbegi,
who should be following me shortly through menopause.*

Contents

✠

Hot Flashes

Introduction

✠

When I had dinner with an old friend recently, I went through the litany of symptoms I had been experiencing over the past few years—the mood swings, hot flashes, night sweats, anxiety attacks—nothing unusual for this time of my life. Overjoyed to find a companion sufferer, my friend began to divulge all the symptoms she had been dealing with over the past several years—in ignorance of their cause. When she tried to tell her doctor what she was experiencing, he pooh-poohed her concerns, told her there was nothing wrong with her, *and never mentioned menopause as a possible cause of her troubles.* She thus feared heart attack, brain tumor, cancer—as various parts of her body responded to the hormonal havoc in her system.

My friend works with Alzheimer's patients, and thus was truly frightened when she noticed her own memory failing her more and more often. Was she in the beginning stages of this disease? The final embarrassment for this religious and chaste single woman was a sudden lust that engulfed her in the presence of any male. Was she going crazy? And would these feelings last the rest of her days? For years my friend suffered in ignorance.

At dinner that night, we had a great time sharing our stories. It was comforting to know someone else was going through a similar process, and that there might be some relief for our suffering. Later I realized that I had never asked my friend—the times I'd seen her over the past few years—if she was going through menopause. This should have been a natural question since I was going through it myself and my friend is exactly my age. But in our culture, asking a woman if she's going through menopause is considered impolite, like asking her if she's had a face-lift or dyed the gray in her hair. Any suggestion that a woman is aging is auto-matically an insult.

Our youth-worshipping culture has no place for old women. That makes our menopausal burden even heavier than it might be. Social and cultural factors play a critical role in women's climacteric experience. Bio-logical factors alone do not explain everything. In fact, keeping up with all the medical studies on menopause still leaves us without clear answers or solutions.

For me, sharing stories with other women going through "the Change" gave me a community of sister travelers—a place where we shared com-fort, information, and encouragement to persevere in our search for answers and relief. I found these women on an Internet discussion group, and was astounded by the variety and sameness of their stories, the com-passion and helpfulness of their comments to each other. A new member wrote, "I'm soon to be forty-eight, haven't had a period in almost two years, and most of the time I feel I could bite a nail in two—but by read-ing your notes, I now realize I'm not losing my mind or turning into the insomniac bitch from hell." When another member told about her gyne-cologist demanding that she continue to take a medication that made her miserable, we all told her to find a new gyn. She finally heeded the advice, and is now feeling much better under the care of a different doctor.

When new women join our Internet group, they invariably say how helpful it is to hear other women's stories. It is a nourishment they were famished for, these personal narratives that tell the tale of an individual, but also of the universal passage through the Change of Life. It doesn't matter if we've heard a particular story before. As Janet Burroway says, "True stories are only believed with frequent telling."

We need to hear other women's stories, and we can't always get them from our families. "This wasn't something I could have asked my mother about," writes Sara McAulay, "even assuming she hadn't died years earlier. I couldn't have asked her, or any of my aunts or female cousins either. To hear most of them tell (or not tell) it, they'd never *had* sex, at least not in living memory. Vaginal discomfort? To hear them tell (or not tell) it, none of them owned a vagina of any description, let alone one in which dryness might qualify as a change worth remarking."

Mary Swander found herself without a female support system either, until the day a friend sent two women over to clean her house. Mary had been hemorrhaging for three weeks—"weak and dizzy, my hands and feet blue"—and in exhausted desperation, accepted this help. As the women worked, they shared their own menopause stories. "Here were my sisters educating me about the sequence of the events to come in my body." It is this sharing that brings us back into community, that reassures us we are not going crazy or dying, but passing through a normal stage of life.

Another reason our stories must be told again and again is to destroy the taboo that surrounds the topic of menopause. When another woman mentions her heavy bleeding, Mary Swander nods in embarrassment, "for the topic was one that made me and everyone else I knew—both men and women, acquaintances and close friends alike—very uncomfortable." Sue Walker, teaching a class on Aging and Literature, finds that when she starts to discuss an essay on menopause with her class, "I feel like I have peanut butter stuck to the roof of my mouth." I wonder, as I read Sue Walker's essay, whether I would have the courage to discuss menopause with my own classes. It is bad enough, I think, that my face and neck turn beet red periodically for no apparent reason, that beads of sweat accumulate on my brow. My students can probably tell by looking at me.

This is what a gynecologist told me at the end of my forty-eighth year: "I can tell by looking at you that you're menopausal. There's no need to do blood tests." Of course, she meant she could tell by examining my vagina, but for me the phrase stuck. "I can tell by looking at you."

Is the world able to tell by looking at me?

This same gynecologist told me to keep taking Premarin although I was experiencing side effects of awful depression and rage, "unless you are going to put a bullet in your head." Such statements, unfortunately, are too common. When Sue Walker refused hormones, her doctor "stooped over, staggered a few feet and asked: 'Do you want to be one of those little old humped-backed ladies on elevators?'" After a lengthy bout of bleeding, Janet Burroway went to a new gyn who told her, "I'm certainly going to take your womb out," and when she protested, he insisted, "I'm the doctor."

The medical model, as anthropologist Denise Spitzer points out, "defines menopause as an endocrine deficiency disease analogous to diabetes; thus menopause is regarded as a pathology which requires medical intervention. In the medical literature, menopausal women are often portrayed not just as aging, but decaying." In *The Change*, Germaine Greer critiques this medical prescription:

The medicalization of menopause is the last phase in the process of turning all the elements of female personality that do not relate to the adult male into pathology. Virginity is pathology; lack of interest in heterosexual intercourse on demand is pathology; 'excessive' involvement in mothering is pathology; middle-aged truculence and recalcitrance are the most pathological of all. Now we have pills for all of them and women are obediently taking them.

We require an interpretation of menopause that goes beyond the medical model—beyond pathology. And who might better show us the rich possibilities of what this passage means than women writers on their own experience? For some, it means facing the loss of self—that feeling of being estranged, alienated, displaced from our center. Who is this person inhabiting my body? Moody, forgetful, weepy, and ranting, she scares me as she chases away my friends and loved ones. And what is this body that I can no longer recognize as mine? Thickening, slowing, heating up and freezing, awake or sleepy round the clock, growing hair where it shouldn't—losing what it had, bleeding for weeks in a row or not at all, lusting obsessively or losing libido along with its juice; slackening skin, moles, brown spots, and skin tags, fibroids and assorted lumps, bladder malfunction, constipation, weak eyes, brittle bones. What is this body trying to tell me?

The losses are abundant, specific, and palpable. Catherine Reid writes of "wondering where all the blood is going to go. Not the monthly period blood, because I'll be glad when the last trace is finally gone, but the blood that has been in my poems and dreams." Sue Walker states it bluntly as "the cessation of blood and all that means: a figure going to hell, breasts sagging, back aches, the threat of lung disease, heart disease, cancer." And for some, blood does not stop without a raging torrent preceding the cessation.

One loss exacerbated by a culture that worships youth and beauty is the loss of that admiration for our physical selves. "I was accustomed to men looking at me," reflects Norma Fox Mazer. "Now men don't look at me much anymore. . . . and I miss it." Marilyn Krysl admits, "I miss myself as a calendar girl, and at times I still feel sadness for this loss." Krysl reports that when she told a male friend she had been invited to write about menopause, he said, "'a compliment to your writing ability, but not to your youth and beauty.'"

It is the fear of what we might become that is probably the worst. Sara McAulay tells about "the horror stories I'd heard all my life. . . . I'd have night sweats and mood swings; I'd become what the men in my ex-husband's family called a 'Menopause Minnie'—shrill and irrational, sexless, unattractive. My cunt would dry up. I'd grow a beard." The monster's breath is particularly hot on our necks when we fear the menopausal experiences of our mothers, aunts, and grandmothers. When McAulay was a young girl, she feared her mother was dying while hemorrhaging and could think of no way to help her. Mary Robertson remembers an Arkansas childhood where women were likely to lose their minds when they reached the "change":

> There was one mad woman I never heard talked about when I was a child, perhaps because she died before I was born. I didn't know until I was grown that my own grandmother, my father's mother, was one of those who lost her mind at the 'change,' going into a depression that refused to lift. One fine summer morning she got out of bed before anyone else in the house was awake, went to the kitchen, and drank some of the lye kept under the sink for making hominy. It took her a week to die.

Gloria Steinem reports that the first stage of dealing with aging for her was denial. "I was going to continue living *exactly as I always had*—and make a virtue of it. If age were ever to interrupt sexual life, for instance, I would just continue it in a different way. After all, the world could use a pioneer dirty old lady." Sara McAuley writes that the fear was not of aging and death, but of becoming invisible:

> I was afraid of the loss of color and energy of all kinds; the leaching away of wildness and juice and smoke and the ability to travel light and the willingness to do so at a moment's notice. I was afraid not so much of growing old or dying as of growing timid and tame.

For many of us, menopause is a signal that our days are numbered. Or as Ellen Gilchrist more eloquently puts it, "You have been reminded of mortality and death and where you are in space and time." Heading down the other side of the slope of our lives, we wonder if we will live to do the things we've dreamed of, or ever fulfill the aspirations of our youth. Faye Moskowitz reflects, "I wonder if I have time left to write a novel; will I ever shape the hoarded bits of brightly colored fabric into the quilt I have always thought I'd make one day?" Mary Robertson reports, "It seemed to me that opportunities and possibilities were closing down. . . . At two-thirty in the morning when my eyes suddenly opened I saw myself on a downward slide that would end only with my death."

Yet this closing down, this interview with mortality, when faced and embraced—leads to a richer or as rich a life, although a changed one. Robertson finally sees that "if we don't accept change in our lives then we start to die, and I wasn't ready to do that just yet. Having passed through one change in my life, I was ready to move on to the next." Cecelia Holland speaks of a similar transition: "I had come through something. I had endured a transforming fire. I was ready for what came next."

Cultural attitudes play a significant part in women's menopausal experience. Denise Spitzer reports after studying ninety-six cultures that "role change—or shifts in the expected or anticipated activities or responsibilities of women" was one of the key factors across cultures in how women experience menopause. She points out that changes occur temporally, also. "In North America, for example, the symptoms of menopause now include osteoporosis and vaginal atrophy whereas formerly involutional melancholia and digestive problems were the predominant symptoms."

In her interpretation and teaching of Virginia Woolf's *To the Lighthouse*, Bonnie Braendlin says she always identified with the character of Lily Briscoe "as a representation of the early twentieth-century 'New Woman' artist," rather than with the older dedicated wife and mother of eight, Mrs. Ramsey. "I suddenly realized that Mrs. Ramsey . . . at fifty, was I—or rather, I was identifying with *her*—and we were both *menopausal women*, an epithet, a concept, and a subject position more denigrated and resisted in my culture than the Angel in the House was in Woolf's. . . . In a (hot) flash I shifted my interpretive interest from Lily to Mrs. Ramsey."

The fifty-plus woman in North American culture is invisible. It is no wonder, then, that we feel we are disappearing at menopause. "Within this country," writes Gloria Steinem, "African-American women reported the fewest negative symptoms and Jewish women reported the most; arguably because of the relative importance of the role that older women play in those communities."

In essay after essay, women face the cultural stereotype that would pin them to the wall. Marilyn Krysl paints this portrait in stark reality:

> Here in twentieth-century America old women are perceived not only as superfluous but distinctly in the way. They are sterile, useless, ugly: an insult to the economy. Only the childish granny threatens no one, but even this harmless creature is barely tolerated. The young are socialized to view old women as a drag on their thoughtlessness, a blight on the landscape of chic decadence and turn-on sexuality hyped by pornography.

For me, it was the internalization of this portrait that made facing my aging so painful. I had always believed the stereotype. I myself was not interested in old women. I thought them irrelevant. How, then, could I become one?

The old woman I knew best as a child was my grandmother—a lump of useless flesh—dumpy, grim, contributing nothing. She and I sometimes had to sleep in the same bed, and I was afraid of being contaminated by her. She complained. She sat around on Saturdays (her sabbath as a Seventh Day Adventist) and let my mother wait on her. I felt the intense sense of duty emanating from my mother, along with the resentment and lack of affection. Grandma was an object to be scorned and ridiculed. Her religion did not allow her to eat pork, but she greedily asked for second helpings of my mother's famous stuffing—made with pork, of course. We all had a good laugh at Grandma's expense.

This scenario could have been different. My grandmother was a talented woman. She had been an expert seamstress and in her later years made paper flowers so delicate and lifelike, they rivalled those fresh from the garden. She spent hours teaching me her craft, yet I felt no joy or gratitude. In my household, paper flowers were ridiculed and to this day I cannot appreciate them. They represent the dry, juiceless imitation of life—the old, withered thing that was my grandmother.

It is this old, withered thing that I fear becoming myself. When I read the phrase "a fifty-year-old woman" in a short story or novel, everything it conjures up congeals and tightens in my stomach. Why, I want to know, is there not a positive literary portrayal of the older woman? Of menopause itself?

I wanted to do this book to provide a literary forum for menopause, as well as to explore the diversity of women's experiences. I wanted to help break the taboo of silence, of shame, of modesty. And most of all, I wanted to offer readers the solace, understanding, and confidence that comes from hearing other women's stories. We are not alone. We are not suffering in isolation. There is a pattern. There are alternatives. There is meaning in our menopausal experience.

MARY SWANDER

The Cleaning Woman Rag

✠

With mops, brooms and buckets in hand, Shirley and Marlane pushed open my back door and wound their way, clanking and banging, up the narrow flight of steps into my kitchen.

"Your friend Fran sent us over. Said you needed a little help over here. Is this the right place?" they asked. "Are you Mary?"

I welcomed the pair inside and immediately they set to work. Shirley, the tall, thin member of the duo, dressed in tight fitting jeans and a sweat shirt, shook scouring powder into the sink, her blond wig bobbing with the rhythm of the movement of her hands rubbing the sponge across the stainless steel. Marlane, short and plump, her flowered pedal pushers creeping up toward her knees, uncoiled the cord of the vacuum cleaner and with a tap of her fist, knocked the hardwood floor attachment into place.

"Where's the plug?" Marlane asked.

"Just behind that door," I said. "You can skip my study. I'll be work-ing in that room, and will clean it later myself."

"Fine," Shirley nodded without even looking up. "Have you got some extra rags?"

"Oh, here's the plug."

"I have plenty of rags."

"Another professor," Marlane said.

"Must be writing a book," Shirley said.

"Yup, they's all writing books."

I pulled part of an old flannel pajama top out of the rag bag in my closet, then retired to my study, where I closed the door and tried to plunge into a stack of student papers. After grading three of them, I put

8

my head down on my desk and cried in exhaustion, tearful but inaudible sobs that would not draw the attention of the cleaning women. I had never before had anyone clean my house. The whole idea seemed too classist, elitist and costly, but after I had been coping with three weeks of menopausal hemorrhaging, I finally gave in and accepted Fran's gift.

I was teaching at a major midwestern university and it was close to finals—a critical point in the semester. Weak and dizzy, my hands and feet blue, my hemoglobin count down to seven (normal is around twelve), I had been shuffling to campus to attempt to teach my classes, only to come home again to collapse into bed. Now, I was glad to have some help, someone out there in my house tidying up the place. For a moment, when I heard the buzz and whir of the vacuum cleaner in the living room, I felt more in control. Yet when I glanced at the stacks of papers and reports piled up in front of me, I didn't know how I would ever be able to finish the term. What's more, the three different doctors I had consulted in the past three years seemed blasé about my condition.

"Oh, yes. Hemorrhaging is a common problem," they all said.

"You're in menopause," my gynecologist told me on the phone when my problems first began. He didn't even examine me.

"Menopause? At forty?"

"Yes, well you're in mini-menopause. You'll bleed like this now when you're forty, then again when you're fifty."

"Mini-menopause?" I questioned my GP.

"Never heard of such a thing," he said. "You're clearly in menopause. Should be almost finished with it soon. Maybe another year."

"I want to know how far I'm along in menopause," I asked yet another gynecologist I consulted. "I can't wait to be finished."

"Finished? You haven't even started," he said.

A knock on the door roused me, and Shirley entered the room. We stared at each other for a moment in silence, she noting the tears on my cheeks, me feeling an enormous lethargy and inertia in my chair. I thought she needed more cleaning materials and I wondered if I could just direct her to them rather than having to find them myself.

"Fran told us you was having the heavy bleeding," she said from the doorway.

I nodded in embarrassment, for the topic was one that made me and everyone else I knew—both men and women, acquaintances and close friends alike—very uncomfortable.

"Well, Marlane had the same thing," Shirley said. "We thought you might want to come out and hear about her deal."

Suddenly, here was a woman talking very directly to me about menopause with an ease I hadn't experienced in my university colleagues. During the previous two years, I had tried not to mention my problem to my friends. Whenever I did, a blush came over their faces and mine, and then we fell into awkwardness. So instead, I plowed along, teaching my classes, seeing my students, attending my committee meetings, feeling all the time that my very life force was draining out of me.

In our Western culture, menstrual blood has always been taboo. The Old Testament speaks of menstruating women as "unclean," and for ten centuries' worth of Christianity, menstruating women were forbidden to come to church. In ancient patriarchal societies around the world, women were shunned and sent to menstrual huts once a month, until their purification process was complete. In contemporary culture, menstruating women do the opposite, but with the same amount of shame. They function through their lives, putting on the facade that nothing is happening. From adolescence onward, we worry that a spot might show, that we will give ourselves away by our odors. The higher up the ladder of social sophistication we are, the less we talk about these things.

We lead our lives in isolation, one woman to one nuclear family, rarely discussing or acknowledging—certainly never celebrating—these great changes that go on in our bodies, these biological rhythms that keep us attuned to the forces of the universe, the lunar calendar, the rising and falling of the tides. Seldom do we stop and feel a sense of belonging, one with the other, or acknowledge that when we bleed, we are carrying a sacredness within us, an ability to create life, to continue the mystery of the propagation of the species, to continue the mystery of all existence. And when something "goes wrong," when we suffer from horrible cramps, or are hemorrhaging, we feel silenced and stuck with our "flaw."

I followed Shirley into the kitchen. Yes, I thought, inching along, my hands bracing me on the walls as I teetered through the hallway, I would love to hear about another woman's menopausal experience. Any experience, whether similar to mine or not. I was forty-two years old and few of my friends—even those who were fifty—had entered menopause. For three years, I had been on this journey alone, without feedback or a measure to go by. I had found a couple of books on the subject, but a mere paragraph or two had been devoted to my problem, and the concluding sentences always cut off with the abrupt solution: "A hysterectomy is the usual prescribed course of action." A terrifying and invasive procedure, a life threatening procedure for someone like me who was allergic to all kinds of anesthetics. No, I thought, I wasn't happy that another woman had suffered as I had, but yes, I was comforted to know that someone else had gotten through to the other side. Intact.

I slumped down at the table, and Shirley swept up the food crumbs with the broom.

"I'm really sorry for the mess," I said.

"Oh, we've seen mess," Shirley said.

"The cats have shed all over the porch. I'll put them in their box before you clean out there."

"Don't worry about it," Shirley said. "We've handled cats before."

"And dogs," Marlane said. "Oh, them dogs of Fran's."

"Now, them little ones ain't so bad."

"But that Great Dane!"

"Knocks the plates right off the kitchen table with one swish of its tail."

"All the professors got dogs."

"Least two."

"Sometimes even three or four."

"Just like their computers. One in every room."

"Yup, they love their dogs."

"Naw, we've handled dogs and cats before," Shirley said. "And gerbils."

"And ferrets," Marlane added.

"And boa constrictors."

"Clean out a boa constrictor cage, now that's a mess," Marlane said. She filled a bucket with hot water in the sink, suds floating over the rim. "Oh boy, we've cleaned up messes you would not believe."

"Now, as for your mess," Shirley said. "Marlane done the same thing as you."

"Yup," Marlane said, plunging the mop into the bucket and bending down to wring out the sponge. "I had the bleeding real bad. I'd go for a month and nothing. Then another month and nothing. Then *whosh!*" From the mop head, water gushed back into the pail.

"Yeah," Shirley said. "She'd get so weak she could hardly stand. Kind of drunk like. Just like you. She'd be weaving around. And finally she couldn't work. I had to zoom around twice as fast to keep up with our regular houses."

"How long did this go on?" I asked.

"Oh, about eighteen months."

"I've been doing this much longer than that."

"Well," Shirley said, "every woman's different. That's the thing. No one's alike. You just got to get rid of the idea that you'll do like another woman." She dumped the dustpan full of crumbs into the garbage. "It helps to know about other women, sure, but you can't go by it exactly. Better to go by your mother. You do pretty much what she did. What did your mother do?"

What did my mother do? I couldn't really remember. My mother, who died when I was twenty-three, did hemorrhage, but that was about all I knew of her menopause. I had tried to do the math in my head. When I was fifteen, she was fifty, I remember coming home from school one spring day and finding her lying on the couch, her skin the same color as the blue paisley slipcover, her feet propped up with pillows.

"I'm hemorrhaging," she had said quietly and calmly in response to my look of panic at discovering her in such a condition. She picked up on my anxiety immediately, the worries of a young girl who had just begun to enter womanhood. "Sometimes this happens to women in menopause," she said, then quickly added, "but it doesn't necessarily mean it will happen to you."

How many times did that happen to her? In how many years? I couldn't piece it together. I knew there were enough rounds of bleeding to require a trip to the hospital and a D&C. I knew there was talk of a possible hysterectomy. I knew there were embarrassing stains on some of her clothes.

"Do you think you can get this stain out?" I remember her handing one of her best dresses to the laundry man, a red blotch marring the beautiful white silk.

I stood there on the landing of the stairway and in my adolescent shyness, could not believe my mother could even show a man that dress. I would have wadded it up and thrown it away.

"Oh," he laughed. "That's nothing. That'll be easy to remove. A couple of weeks ago, a woman up the block gave me a dress that was completely soaked in blood, and we got it cleaned up for her. I mean it was completely soaked."

Had the woman been shot? I thought. Good grief, a woman just a few blocks away had been covered with blood, a neighbor had suffered an assault, and no one had been told. Had she been stabbed? Why hadn't this been in the papers? No, from the look my mother gave the laundry man when she handed over the other dry cleaning—my father's suits, a couple of my brothers' sweaters—I finally understood that this neighbor woman had been hemorrhaging, too. The laundry man was actually expressing a kind of sympathy and understanding for my mother and her menopausal situation by telling her about something even worse. All this in a strange adult code. At fifteen, I found the adult world a strange and confusing place.

At forty-two, I didn't find it that different. Without my mother there as a guide or role model, without her there to offer encouragement or support, to pass on her experience and wisdom, I was adrift in the patriarchal world of conventional medicine. I had no sisters. Both my parents had been only children, so I had no cousins or aunts. Both my grandmothers were also dead. What I needed was a tribe, a matriarchy of women to gather around me and inform me about this magical rite that I was going through, this passage that linked a woman to women of every size, race and culture through all time.

Again, I swept through my mind for the crumbs of tribal memory that might be useful. When I was a young child, my mother and grandmother used to load me in the car and drive twenty miles to the county seat to shop and visit with the members of our extended family—my grandmother's siblings and their children, spouses and grandchildren. These were weekday visits, and often all the women would congregate at one house to consolidate efforts for my aging grandmother. The women sat in hardback chairs, coffee cups and sugar cookies strewn across the kitchen table, and traded gossip and folk wisdom.

"Mabel's pregnant again."

"Oh, oh . . ."

"They do come along."

"You put a mustard pack on that knee."

"Will that work?"

"See if it don't."

Elliptical, their conversation drifted from sex to arthritis, from the personal to the painful, the emotional to the physical. Theirs was a much more complicated code than the laundry man's. Theirs was a language of metaphor, of synecdoche, and connotation blurring together, weaving in and out like the braids of my grandmother's hair—the poetry of a private women's knowledge.

"Hope it's okay."

"Mercy."

"At forty-four?"

"Drains the water right off."

"Mercy. That can happen."

"You put the pack directly on the knee?"

"Well, wrap it in a towel."

"She thought she was finished, see."

"Then toot-toot, along comes a caboose."

I was seven, and the talk was boring and put me in a stupor. Trained not to whine, I played with the spoon in the sugar bowl or leaned my head onto my mother's shoulder and went to sleep.

But now, when I rewind the tapes in my head, I realize that my tribe was actually initiating me into the workings of womanhood. Without using language like PMS, PPD or menopause, they understood the workings of the female body.

"Wish I could drain the water off elsewhere."

"She going to take a dive again when she has this one?"

"Hope not."

"Oh yeah, the water. Makes you so cross."

"So cross."

"You got to get that old water off."

"Watermelon."

"Watermelon?"

"Eat lots of it. Drink the seeds as a tea."

"She's had such a time with that. Mercy."

"That'll do it?"

"You bet."

How I longed for these women to gather once again, to enter my house and sip a cup of coffee and find a solution for me. How I longed to join an even more primitive circle of council, all of us sitting on the ground, rocking and swaying in unison, the priestesses or wise women there to offer guidance and healing. Just when I needed them the most, I found myself without a female support system of any kind. Or had I?

"Yup, then that bleeding stopped one day. Just stopped. Finally stopped," Marlane said. With a powerful grip on her hand, she yanked up the lever that wrang out the mop head. Water spurted from the sponge. Marlane jerked the lever again and again. One final droplet of water plopped into the bucket. She leaned the mop in the corner of the kitchen and picked up the Windex, spritzing the dining room window.

"Then watch out," Marlane said. "Just as soon as that stops, you get the hot flashes. And boy, the sweat just pours off you." Beads of the spray rolled down the window. With three quick movements of her hand, Marlane smeared the chemical across the glass, then with the squeegee forced the water to trickle toward the sill. Dry, the glass sparkled, the early morning May light flooding through and casting a soft yellow glow over the dining room table.

Here were my sisters, my two priestesses engaged in domestic ritual, educating me about the sequence of the events to come in my body. How strange, I thought, that I was so unprepared for this end of the menstrual spectrum. As an adolescent, I was overprepared for the onset of menses. I began menstruating just after my twelfth birthday, but just after my eleventh, my mother kicked into gear. She explained the process to me, gave me a book with even more explicit sexual information and set up a little packet complete with pad and belt in the bathroom closet.

"When the time comes—" she said, "and it will be soon, maybe in a month or two—you'll have these things here when you need them."

Two months passed, and nothing.

"Has the time come yet?" my mother asked offhandedly one night when we were doing dishes at the kitchen sink.

I shook my head, and two more months passed.

"Has the time come yet?" she inquired again.

More months passed, and she gave me a refresher course on the intricacies of managing a period. I was prepared. I was so prepared that I was beginning to think the whole thing was a hoax.

Certainly, I've heard tales of all sorts of young girls who were completely left without any information around the beginning of menarche, and although my preparedness may have been extreme, most of my peers seem to have gone through a somewhat similarly enlightened initiation. But where is the information, the education, the comforting nod at the kitchen sink on the other end of the experience? Menstruation is a taboo subject no matter which way you examine it, but why is menopause so much more hush-hush? Even for women who still have their mothers to help them through?

Is it the medical system that reduces menopause to a list of "symptoms"? *Harrison's Principles of Internal Medicine*, one of the most widely read medical textbooks, describes menopause like this:

> The menopause is defined as the final episode of menstrual bleeding in women. . . . During this period there is gradual progressive loss of ovarian function and a variety of endocrine, somatic, and psychological changes. . . . The most common menopausal symptoms are those of the vasomotor instability (hot flush), atrophy of the urogenital epithelium and skin, decreased breast size, and osteoporosis.

Or is it our societal attitude toward aging? Menarche, even with all its taboos, still equals fertility, production, a woman becoming sexually developed and available. Menopause equals the opposite. And in our culture, when a woman's sexual worth is no longer, she is no longer. No wonder there's been so little written, so little researched on the topic. Where's the value? What's the point?

The point is that women should celebrate this transitional time, one with another, gathering together to acknowledge a passage into another phase of life—one filled with more clarity, independence and wisdom. Women should also go off by themselves, rest, play, sing, dance, meditate and pray. Women should stop, stay very still and value themselves, take stock of past accomplishments, achievements and project future successes. In the larger scope of things, women should find menopause a time of contentment—a time to grieve old losses and sorrows, yes, but also a time to let go of the pressures to fulfill others' needs and expectations.

Instead, we struggle along, coping with pathology alone. And what are women left with? For the baby boomer generation, a few more books, a few more resources than were available a generation ago. For the lucky ones, a tribe that will surround and support them with folk wisdom. But for the rest of us, perhaps the fortunate sharing of our experience, older woman to younger, one with another, as we mop the floor.

"Have you got more of them rags?" Shirley asked, down on her knees, scrubbing the baseboards. "I'm going to need more rags."

I fished in the closet and brought out the whole rag bag. On the top were my old pajama bottoms. I handed them to Shirley.

"You ain't been flashing yet?" Marlane asked. She spritzed another window.

"No, no hot flashes so far," I said.

"You will," Marlane said. "Be prepared. Oh, boy."

"Now, some don't get them so bad," Shirley said.

"You haven't had them?" I asked Shirley.

"No, I'm fifty and haven't even started," Shirley said.

"And I'm forty-eight," Marlane huffed. "And I'm finished. What a woman don't go through."

"Have you got a rag smaller than this?" Shirley asked, holding up the pajama bottoms.

"Oh, go ahead and just rip that up," I said.

"Now, who's your doctor, honey?" Marlane asked.

"Dr. Crook."

"Crook?"

"At the hospital?"

"Yes."

"She's doctoring with Crook at the hospital," Marlane repeated to

Shirley, who was attempting to make a small tear in the pajama bottoms with her teeth.

"Well, that's part of your problem," Shirley said. "Got to get you a woman doctor."

"When did a man ever go through menopause?" Marlane asked. "Now, you know . . ." She stopped and yanked the attachment off the end of the vacuum cleaner hose. "They can go up there and suck it all out."

"Get you a woman doctor," Shirley insisted. She pulled a large pair of scissors from the kitchen drawer. "Not so happy with the knife, if you know what I mean?" Shears in hand, she made a large incision in the crotch of the pajama bottoms. "Here, take this side," she told Marlane, tossing one pant-leg to her partner. "Now pull." With perfectly orchestrated precision, the two women leaned in opposite directions, the flannel giving way with a pop and rip, the cotton unraveling, threads dangling, the legs dividing into two separate parts.

"What a woman don't go through."

MARILYN KRYSL

To Live Intentionally, to Live Deliberately...

In my daydream I walk uphill, through forest, then emerge into a clearing. The meadow is wide, rambling, sunlit, sprinkled with wildflowers and short grasses. The air is mild. Birds flitter in the trees at the edge, and I lie down in the sun. The grass has a dry tang mixed with intimations of humus and the mild perfume of small flowers. I'm alone because I've come here to do what only I can do, alone. This is the landscape of my death.

In my mid-forties this daydream came to me again and again. It would bloom while I walked to work, folded laundry or put away books, sweaters, shoes. It would come while I cooked or raked leaves. I embraced it, indulged it, made it my companion, hoping to load the dice in my favor. For we aren't free to choose the place of our death the way animals do, when they leave their fellows and go off by themselves. Did I hope to nudge my guides and gods? Here's a graceful and beautiful way it might happen. Help me find this.

The daydream was also preparation for menopause. I'd thought of menopause as loss, a death of part of me. I'd anticipated it for a decade. For better or worse it would be a transformation, and I wanted to be conscious, to lean into it, to go with its motion, gracefully. I hoped it would be informed by the beauty of my daydream. But the dream was romantic, cut off from the reality in which I live. For here in twentieth-century America old women are perceived not only as superfluous but distinctly in the way. They are sterile, useless, ugly: an insult to the economy. Only the childish granny threatens no one, but even this harmless creature is barely tolerated. The young are socialized to view old women as a drag on their thoughtlessness, a blight on the landscape of chic decadence and turn-on sexuality hyped by pornography.

I remembered my grandmother, who'd been uprooted from her wheat farm to live the last twenty of her ninety-nine years on the coast with my parents, in unfamiliar surroundings, cut off from a lifetime's worth of friendships. My parents loved her, but they worked. They lived in an isolated suburb, and my grandmother had no way to be out and about. She'd spent those years utterly alone, and I'd contributed to her loneliness. I was adolescent, and I'd bought the myths about old women. I threw away this blood relative who once had been my soulmate as though she were a dirty rag. I took up with fashion, the goddess Sophistication, graduate school, marriage, and Beauty as prescribed by Madison Avenue. I cultivated denial: What had happened to her would not happen to me.

The culture suggests an antidote against demons: plastic surgery. In my forties the idea attached itself to my psyche like a burr. I *knew* the perception of old women as ugly was used to manipulate women into consuming cosmetics and risking surgery, and I was irritated: My imagination was supposed to be *mine*, inviolable and private. Now images of the young and gorgeous invaded, female terrorists in black leather jackets, red lipstick, Terminator glasses. They crowded in, Sirens of trivia and illusion, clamoring with screechy voices, desecrating my space, using up my energies. The surgeon in his green gown smiled and did not mention his fee: He merely wanted to be "helpful."

All right, I decided to just go ahead and imagine it. I called up the things I heard about surgery: pain, swelling, bruises, a long, uncomfortable convalescence inside a plaster helmet. It sounded like mutilation. And it was shameful: You were supposed to sneak away, say you were off to Cuernevaca for some sun. Worse was imagining afterward. I'd have a face which objectively might be called "attractive." But *attractive* is a dubious word, in this instance implying life without soul or juiciness: Would my face resemble a mask, all nuance gone, Nancy Reagan forever? Most sobering was the story of a friend's aunt whose surgeon had botched the job. The skin of her face was pulled back too tightly. She endured for a while in pain, then murdered her surgeon, committed suicide.

But something even more vital topped these considerations. Plastic surgery would be a violation of me, my history, my being in the world. My integrity.

My periods were becoming irregular, diminishing. Menopause was on the way. Eventually I'd have to face those nasty cultural perceptions: ugliness, uselessness, sterility. Invisibility. Why not get it over with? Why not invite these Furies over? Everybody wants a hearing, and I wanted them where I could see them. I sent invitations, rolled out the red carpet. They came in their Porsches, the men with beepers, the women in clattering high heels. I poured white wine, served cappuccino and smiled. The women performed their can-can in a chorus line, jabbed pins into their dolls, pulled each other's hair. The men smoked and casually knifed each other in the back. A few banged the table or stood to deliver the obligatory old boy line.

I endured their shrillness, the droning boredom of their small minds, their cattiness, the passive-aggressive double entendres. A moment came then when everyone fell silent. They'd gone through their repertoire, run down. One by one they mashed their cigarettes and without another word walked out. Occasionally I see one of them from a distance, but they keep to the other side of the street.

I have wanted living to be an aesthetic act. I visualized moving into menopause as a forward and upward motion, the slow, gradual ascending of an eagle or a swan with a strong body and huge wings climbing to a height where she can soar. But to ascend you have to let go, and I didn't want to, not yet. I liked my periods. I liked being the proud bearer of a built-in body calendar. I didn't need a watch or daily planner. I felt rather than merely noted the passage of time: Its moments passed through me, as I passed through them. And I liked the monthly repetition of a pattern. For a week after my period I'd feel as though I'd just emerged from a chrysalis. My wings were drying. Then fluids began to collect in me, my breasts began to swell. For about ten days before my next period I'd feel especially desirous, desirable. Bleeding was a climax, a celebration: Now the month's spiral with all its little idiosyncrasies belonged to me. I'd made it mine. The cyclic was in me down to the very bone.

It wasn't easy to give up something so intimately part of my identity. My letting go began with a late spring snow. I'd been bleeding less, and the color of the blood was darker. The crab apple blossoms had come out, and the air was warm. Now this wet snow. It would melt by morning. Falling now, it seemed an emblem of impermanence. And that evening, while I watched this snow drift down, I received news of two deaths: of a child of one of my daughter's friends, and, a few minutes later, of the death, in India, of a woman friend who was only fifty.

I was alone in the house. Though the flakes were wet, there was a delicacy about them. I thought of my daughter who, when she says good-bye, walks a few steps, then turns and waves again, as though she can't quite resign herself to going. Suddenly I was crying. I cried slowly, deeply, and for a long time. For I was mourning more than those deaths. I mourned the end of a season, the end of my daughter's childhood, the end of child-bearing. Afterward, I experienced that calm emptiness in which time no longer seems a factor. It's those moments of which Emily Dickinson wrote, "After great pain a formal feeling comes." I heard the drip of runoff from the eave. Good-bye, good-bye.

Good-bye most of all to my body calendar: It had ticked for years, water falling drop by drop on stone. Soon that steady ticking would be gone.

It happens that my menopause, like that of all women of my generation, coincides with a larger, more profound loss. Those of us alive now are wit-nesses to the battering of the planet. No one knows the number of species on earth, even to the nearest magnitude. Estimates vary from five to eighty million, and only about 1.4 million have been even briefly described. Every day between forty and one hundred and forty of these described species disappear. How many species not yet even noticed by human beings are also disappearing?

There'd come a watershed hour in my forties when I'd plumbed the depths of this tragedy. Since then I've been in mourning in the only way that seems appropriate: I try to live as fully as I can, at the same time try-ing not to use more of the planet's resources than I need. Marlo Morgan describes an Aboriginal tribe in Australia that has begun in this genera-tion to practice celibacy. They have been keeping watch for centuries, and now their observations tell them that the web of life on the planet is being irrevocably torn. Their celibacy is deliberate. It's their collective intention to end the life of their group, and, with the death of the last person, to leave the earth.

They've accepted their synchronicity with the planet. In a similar way, to be in menopause now is to be synchronized with this larger death.

My grieving cannot be simply for myself.

In the midst of death what form shall living take? I'd had enough suc-cess at career, enough fulfillment from teaching, plenty of good closeness with friends, the satisfaction of romance, marriage, children. I would go on writing, teaching, loving my children, friends, students. But it was also time to move on. I wanted new work. At the same time I craved more soli-tude. I needed to wander hillside, forest and plain, to listen to the vintage

music of silence. An image from the Persian poet Rumi became important: "Be a full bucket, pulled up from darkness."

I'd experienced this fullness in heightened moments. Now I began to
experience these moments more often. I longed to live, moment by
moment, a life of such fullness.

One advantage I had was writing. There is beauty that has nothing to
do with Madison Avenue, the beauty that characterizes life on earth, and
writing, which addresses this life, is an act of beauty to which William
Carlos Williams's statement about poetry applies: Every day people die
for lack of what is found there. Even if there is ugliness in the subject a
writer addresses, what she articulates about that ugliness has in it the
artist's careful attention to life, the grace of the writing and the beauty
of truth.

Another advantage was the practice of meditation. Meditative attention heightens awareness of beauty and its impermanence. When I sit in
silence, I'm aware of the live world I'm part of. Cleaning a room slowly,
cooking, putting books on shelves, turning compost—the tasks of any
life, done with loving attention, are themselves meditations. But that winter even the compost froze. I decided to spend Sundays volunteering at
the botanical gardens. There, amidst the warmth of sunlight through
glass, I watered, trimmed, potted plants, cleaned the lily tanks and med-
itated Rumi's image.

The next year I finished writing a book and went off for a week's training with Peace Brigade International. PBI began its work in the early
eighties in El Salvador and Guatemala. Volunteers accompany natives of
those countries whose lives are threatened by death squads. The premise
is simple: Death squads are unlikely to try to murder one of their fellow
countrymen while a foreigner is present. Simply escorting someone under
threat will probably save that person's life. In Sri Lanka in 1989 six lawyers
who'd attempted to bring human rights cases to trial had been murdered.
At the invitation of the Sri Lankan Bar Association, PBI volunteers
opened a project in Sri Lanka and began to accompany lawyers and their
clients.

The courage of people like Nobel Peace Prize recipient Rigoberta
Menchu, who risk death by openly defying corrupt governments, has
always astonished me. PBI had accompanied her, and their work seemed
a way to support such people. In April of 1992 I joined the team in Sri
Lanka. I was welcomed as an honorary relative by the families of those I

escorted. This welcome, genuine and spontaneously given, cast our collaboration in intimately human terms. The Roman philosopher Seneca comes close to describing this when he says, "She who does good to another does good also to herself, not only in the consequences but in the very act; for the consciousness of well doing is in itself ample reward." But Seneca's statement, ending with the notion of reward, skews things a bit. St. Francis's prayer is more to the point: It is in giving that we receive.

Those we accompanied suffered tragedy: Their children or relatives had "disappeared" and they themselves might be next. That kind of suffering was not part of my experience. Still, even those like myself, privileged by the fact that we have not suffered those particular tragedies, need to live in a world in which courageous people inspire the rest of us to courageous acts, where together we confront injustice and persevere. The effect of working for PBI was to lift me to a higher level of being. It felt as though I was being pulled up from darkness, and as I rose, being filled.

I began to have hot flashes, but in the sweltering heat of Sri Lanka's summer it hardly mattered. After all, we're made mostly of water. This sweat was just more of the sweat I was sweating anyway, and sweat itself just more of the common humidity. After about three weeks in that climate, it was as though I'd been cleansed of made-in-America, fast-track impurities. My sweat seemed to have become pure water.

Water is healing and the ocean a solitude. When I wasn't escorting clients, I swam out beyond the breakers in the Indian Ocean and floated there in primordial time. The water felt like a huge, kind animal, holding me, rocking. I was busy being reborn.

Witnessing the suffering of the Sri Lankan people reminded me that in the larger scheme of things we're minuscule. By the time I returned to the U.S., menopause seemed just another fact of life. But my culture hadn't changed in my absence. Though my farewell party for the Furies had been a smashing success, no one exorcises them once and for all. When I told a male friend I'd been invited to write about menopause, he said, "A compliment to your writing ability, but not to your youth and beauty." I winced, but his remark didn't carry the sting it might have earlier. For what *had* changed was my perspective on my culture. My dignity as an older woman no longer seemed something the culture could decide or others define for me. I'd define it myself by what I did, how I lived.

I don't want to give the impression that I've "overcome" menopause.

I don't think of menopause as something to be overcome. But I *am* giving myself in good faith to searching out a graceful way through the Big Change. I don't use the word *transformation* as a euphemism for accepting a process over which I have little control. I believe change *is* transformation from one state of being into another. Still, I don't want to trivialize the suffering other women experience by suggesting that community service is the key to controlling night sweats, that gardening will preclude insomnia. Nor do I want to be perceived as associating menopause with the earth's demise in order to aggrandize my personal experience.

I miss myself as a calendar girl, and at times I still feel sadness for this loss. Now my sense of cyclical time is writ not in the chapters of months but in the epic rhythm of a year's seasons. Inside this larger rhythm I continue to be aware of the assault my species mounts against other species and to mourn that great dying. At the same time, out beyond the cycle is what Octavio Paz calls original time, time "which rests on its own infinity." More and more often now I fill like Rumi's bucket, cross over and step into that infinite realm.

I've begun to have a different daydream. I imagine myself neither nun nor monk but an older woman who, along with women and men, engages in contemplation and the daily chores of our small community—cleaning the toilets, weeding the garden, doing laundry, recycling our waste, preparing food. I imagine the day ends with bathing in the women's pool, where we indulge the pleasures of water and talk. We're aware of the great death going on around us, and some of us choose to be celibate. And moment by moment we pay attention to the live world, all of it. We notice both the hawk circling above us and the Christmas trees piled beside a dumpster.

In this daydream events take on a brightness beyond the ordinary, because they're part of a communal life I share with people who know me, and because they take place in a space transformed from the noisy and aggressive violence of everyday life in the U.S.A. I don't yet have the community I've imagined, but I hope gradually to build it in the same way I clean a room or turn the compost. I try to treat my parents, my daughters and my husband with consideration for the stage of life each is in, and when I meet older women now I try to see them, and by seeing to honor who and what they are.

Every day I stand before my grandmother's photograph, and as I study her face, I see her as I couldn't during those years of estrangement. I look in her eyes and ask her to forgive me. Then I go outside and turn some compost, which has been, is and will be a conscious act in which I remember and salute the beautiful, live world. When I do these things with awareness, I am the full bucket pulled up from darkness. Such beautiful choices are my bulwark against the noisy, intractable and intolerant America in which I'm a woman growing older, a woman in the midst of menopause.

CECELIA HOLLAND

Wolftime

⚊

In 1989 I was going crazy. I was forty-five and my head was coming apart.
I screamed at my kids and my lover and wept at nothing. I was a walking catalogue of symptoms. I have always been a little neurotic but it
never bothered me before. Now I felt out of register. I was lost inside an
alien body, monstrous, too large, off-balance. I got dizzy. My hands and
feet tingled a lot. Rushes of nameless horror came over me. One day while
watching a football game I realized that I was about to die, that it was
meaningless even to try to draw breath, and after a moment found myself
sitting there, holding my breath like a woman underwater.

My lover, caught in his own turmoils, seemed to me like an enemy—
an easy enemy, one I could attack with impunity. I bewildered him; he
agreed with me that I was going nuts. Gamely, he held on, but I was
headed for the outer limits.

Two of my daughters were in the virulent stages of adolescence. One
was flunking high school. The other was roaming the streets at night.
My career was on the ropes. I had never had trouble selling my work
before and now suddenly I could sell nothing. I had lost my best contacts
in New York publishing in the purges of the mid-eighties. The whole business was changing; I had actually seen it coming, but ostrich-like had
hoped it would hold off until I had retired, or at least reached a better
position. Instead I was on a steady downward glide. My whole life was
in descent. At night I cruised the small town where I lived, looking for my
errant daughter, and during the day I struggled to finish a novel I had a
contract for but very little interest in.

I fought with my lover constantly. There was something soothing in it,
a sense of power, of real contact I wasn't getting anywhere else. I fright-

ened myself, I felt muffled away in the middle of some fake, a Frankenstein that did things that looked like the things I did, while I watched amazed from a distance. I could feel nothing, not even sadness. Now and then a rush of terror would sweep over me but most of the time I felt only a little breathless, as if I were waiting for something to happen.

I knew something would happen. It couldn't go on like this.

Fighting and screaming and crying, I made it through the rest of that year. I knew I was losing my mind. I couldn't help my children or be kind to my lover. He had his own problems; he could not keep up with mine. I finished the novel, and I took the kids and rented a house in a neighboring town.

In the new house, my oldest daughter moved into her room and shut the door and never came out. The middle one told me she and I had a personality conflict; she would live in her room, going in and out by the window, and I was to avoid her utterly save to give her money. The youngest shuttled back and forth between me and her father, a desperate look on her face.

I sat in my new dining room and read the Durants' *Age of Napoleon*. I could think of nothing to do. I had no life. I had walked out of the old life but had nothing to replace it. One night I dreamt that I was in a house, and a man told me it was haunted by a ghost woman. "What does she do?" I asked. He said, "She sits and reads."

A few days later I went out the back door, and in the alley by the fence my lover was sitting in his car, waiting for me. I got in. We had another fight, but we began seeing each other again. My youngest daughter, who was his child, pressured me to move back in with him. I couldn't do that, but I couldn't give him up, either. For one thing, he fixed my car whenever it broke, and my car was very old and broke a lot. He mowed my lawn and fixed my pipes.

I began to shuttle back and forth between his house and my house; whenever I was with him I wished I was alone; when I was alone I wished I was with him. My oldest daughter had started high school in our new city. After a few months, a teacher she liked said to her, "You know, you could be an A student, but you don't try hard enough." My daughter started bringing books home from school. She started doing homework.

I was seeing my lover nearly every day. My youngest daughter spent most of her time at his house, where she had lived all her twelve years. "It takes a freeway," the Cars sang, "to lead a double life," and I was spending a lot of time on the freeway, going back and forth between the new place and the old place. I bought another house, the biggest house I could find, where I could howl without being heard. I moved into a tiny little room on the top floor, close and dark as a cave. My oldest began liking school now that she was putting something into it. She began getting A's.

My middle girl and I had a fight, in the course of which she hit me with a broom and broke my finger; she was fourteen years old. A few days later she ran away from home to live with her boyfriend. I knew where she was but couldn't talk her into coming back to me. Everybody had advice. Everybody knew I had to get her back somehow. Nobody knew how. My skin crawled all the time. My hands and feet and face tingled. I was shivering apart, coming to pieces, my nerves like rags. I couldn't sleep. At four in the morning I would snap awake as if to a bugle call and lie there knowing everything was terrible and there was nothing I could do about it. Sometimes this feeling developed into actual physical pain, a pressure on all my nerves. If I could get myself up and out of bed I always felt better.

I fired my old agent and hired a new one, but he couldn't sell anything either.

In April of 1992 an earthquake measuring seven Richters hit the county. This did not bother me. Earthquakes are common on the North Coast. This one happened at midday. It toppled whole towns, but they were little towns, and old. I laughed at the rabbity phone calls I got from distant family members. That night as I slept in my cave there was a second violent earthquake at two and a third at four that shook the bed back and forth so hard it knocked against the wall. I began to cry and couldn't stop. I had one kid in the house with me, another twenty miles north in Westhaven, the third twenty miles south in Fortuna with her father. I was drawn and quartered. As soon as it was light I drove down to Fortuna and crawled into bed with my lover and sobbed.

A few nights later, back in the cave, I woke up around one in the morning covered with sweat and hot as a jalapeno. Suddenly, like doors opening, I understood what was happening to me. This was a hot flash. I was going through menopause.

Now I had something to hold on to. This was normal. This would pass. In fact, my oldest daughter seemed to be coming out of her end of the event. She graduated from high school. She went on to the local community college, took algebra, won prizes for her essays. She painted; she made friends. She and I talked about Dickens and read *Great Expectations* together. She explained Greek temples to me so that I understood the menapes and the triglyphs.

I got a job teaching one day a week at a nearby prison, where half my class were murderers. My middle daughter broke up with her boyfriend and came home, somewhat subdued.

I began another novel; if nobody was going to buy it anyway, I could write as I pleased. I left the new agent and went back to the old one, who at least returned my phone calls. She sold some reprint rights. Then she sold an article about my prison job. My middle daughter was sick, had an asthma attack, went into the hospital, lay there as if she were about to die. But she did not die, only ran up a horrendous bill. I went into this trance I go into when I'm hard at work, where the story is playing through my mind like a constant movie and nothing else holds my attention. I had spells of seething lust, followed by spells of utter lack of interest. My periods began to get unpredictable. In the spring I fell into an intense depression that culminated in the collapse of the novel, at about four hundred pages, mostly, I decided now, drivel.

I spent two or three days convinced I would never write again. At night I lay in my bed staring into the dark. During the day I sat around the house drinking coffee and staring out the window. It seemed impossible to move. I ate nothing but candy bars and cookies. After three days I went back to the book and started over. After that, at least, I could sleep.

I tried to focus on what was going on that I liked. My oldest girl was doing very well, working and studying; she claimed to be depressed but she seemed happy enough to me. She had a nice boyfriend. I was getting along very well now with my middle daughter, although she was still flopping around like a bird with a broken wing, sometimes going to school and sometimes not, seemingly heedless of the future. She had a lousy boyfriend. My youngest was showing an alarming tendency to scream and yell and cry. She had been living with her father but when she got her first period she moved back in with me, because she was too embarrassed to ask him to buy Kotex for her. Fortunately, she as yet had no boyfriend.

I still had my teaching job, which I loved; I cared very much for my students, struggling so desperately and valiantly against impossible circumstances. I got another teaching job, this time in an experimental high school, with a whole different array of students, and was amazed that I loved them just as much as the convicts. The pipes under the kitchen sink sprang a leak and I fixed it myself; it was easy. I mowed the lawn. I made fitful attempts at gardening.

I stopped fighting with my lover. In fact, I was no longer interested in my lover in any way, and finally I told him so. He was less crushed than

I had expected. He seemed rather relieved. He asked me if I had another man, and I said no, but he preferred not to believe me.

I had my children, my teaching jobs. I had some interesting friends. The book was going well, too; suddenly it had a shape, a feel, and a forward momentum. It was about as commercial as a three-cup bra, and the current market was for commercial books only, but I thought it was going to be the best novel I had ever written. My periods stopped.

I was liking, more and more, being alone. I began to go to plays and concerts alone, and sometimes to dinner alone, and there was something wildly exciting about it. I felt bigger, somehow, as if now I filled myself out all the way. I belonged to nobody. I was only myself. Oddly, that seemed a wider definition than when I had been mother and lover. I had come through something. I had endured a transforming fire. I was ready for what came next.

GERMAINE GREER

All Your Own Fault

✠

Oppressed women have got rather used to doctors, the only individuals most of them can turn to in time of need, becoming rather testy when faced with problems for which they can find no solution. Many women have given up complaining because of the prevailing response, which implies that really they should just get on with it and stop feeling sorry for themselves. Dr. Mary Anderson, setting forth "the plain facts of the menopause" in a "straightforward, commonsense way" in her book *The Menopause*, might be thought to express the same attitude as the gym mistress who tore up notes to explain that girls had their periods and were to be let off PE.

> It is an interesting reflection that before the menopause became 'popular' I used to advise anxious women who might seek a consultation solely for the purpose of knowing 'what to expect at the menopause' not even to learn to spell the word, far less memorize possible problems. Nowadays such a tritely facetious comment is unacceptable, but the basis for it remains.

What can be the basis for the "facetious comment" if not a poor opinion of women's intellectual abilities? It would be an incurious physician who did not ask, "Why are you worried about it?" Most women who ask what will happen at menopause suspect that they are already experiencing premenopausal symptoms but are reluctant to age themselves by admitting the fact.

The same attitude can be sensed as the basis for Dr. Anderson's confident assertion that two out of three women feel nothing of "any importance to them" during and after the cessation of their periods. Women are only too accustomed to not feeling very well, and are more likely to seek remedies for their children's ailments than their own, which have little "importance to them," but they should not be encouraged in their self-neglect. Traditionally, the medical establishment has given little weight to women's subjective testimony out of an ill-founded conviction that women over-report their symptoms, whereas the case is directly contrary. Menstruation and contraception both affect the quality of women's lives; to many women menopause is just part of a continuum of not-quite-wellness that they accept. *The Menopause*, "a small book . . . for the non-medical reader," produces no proof or even evidence for the statement made on the cover of the first edition that many women pass through this phase of their life "with no effects at all." In their clinics gynecologists usually see only those who complain, and outside a doctor would be unlikely to hear anything about menopause at all. Women don't usually discuss flooding and flushing at dinner parties, and a busy professional like Dr. Anderson probably does not have much time to spend gossiping with the girls.

More insidiously, one statement from *The Menopause* appears to associate lack of menopausal symptoms with sanity, virtue and social status:

> There may be many symptoms and signs associated with the menopause but, especially in the well-balanced, educated, contented woman who finds her family, sexual and professional life fulfilling, *there may be no symptoms whatever.*

These words must have a regrettable knock-on effect upon the woman who has bought a copy of *The Menopause* because she is experiencing symptoms.

Samuel Ashwell, writing in 1844, made the same point, and went on:

> That this does not more constantly happen, arises from the fact, that nature and health are often sacrificed to fashion and luxury . . . habits unwisely begun, and still more unwisely continued.

A hundred years later, though the case had never been proved, the same point was still being made. In 1958 Norton issued a fourth impression of a book by two eminent psychiatrists, O. Spurgeon English, M.D., Professor and Chairman, Department of Psychiatry, Temple University School of Medicine, and Gerald H. J. Pearson, M.D., Dean of the Philadelphia Association for Psychoanalysis. The distressed woman who turns to *Emotional Problems of Living: Avoiding the Neurotic Pattern* for some insight into her climacteric will read this:

> . . . women who have lived unwisely between the ages of twelve and forty-two can build up a great many regrets over which to be irritable, depressed, remorseful, and pessimistic when the menopause appears. . . . Studies of the personalities of those suffering from severe menopause neurosis or psychosis reveal similarities in personality makeup. Such a woman tends to be sensitive and to live a rather isolated social existence. She has not been warm and gregarious, rather one of those women who proudly declare they never visit around much but stay at home and mind their own business. In other words, she has made a virtue of the fact that she was afraid to associate with people or that she did not like people sufficiently to be friendly. Usually she has been strict and pedantic in training her children, often excessively religious, meticulous about cleanliness, many times the excellent housekeeper in whose home no one can be comfortable. She has been sexually frigid, ungenerous and prone to be critical. Such women take little from and give little to the world, so that by the time menopause is reached they not only have no more activity of the sexual glands, but they likewise have become emotionally and spiritually impoverished.

In short, women who suffer at menopause are bad people. In undue fairness, it must be pointed out that this is a picture of the typical sufferer from "severe menopause neurosis or psychosis," and not the typical menopausal female, whereupon it must also be pointed out that no such syndrome as "severe menopause neurosis or psychosis" has been identified. *Clinical* depression is no more common at menopause than in any other epoch of female human life, and the *clinical* depression observed at menopause has no gestures to distinguish it from any other depression. These men, who should be helping the women who trust them, have utterly abandoned their scientific method in order to vilify a kind of woman whom they do not like. They note with satisfaction the high placebo response to the kinds of hormone replacement available in the fifties and go on:

> In a problem of the menopausal syndrome the personality factor that has produced this menopausal symptom should be treated, and the doctor should not depend upon ductless glandular preparations too

much. . . . Women who are not enjoying bringing up their children, who are working too hard and taking life in deadly seriousness, should have it pointed out to them that if they continue this course, they are almost certain to be tired, disillusioned people at fifty.

There is no group of women which has not been identified as courting disaster at menopause. Women who have not exercised their reproductive function in due time have been identified as a specially vulnerable group by some, while others have been equally convinced that women who were excessively attached to their mothering role tend to suffer more. According to Maxine Davis,

> Often busy mothers or energetic careerists who are unwilling or unprepared to acknowledge the termination of the reproductive phase of their lives and the inception of a new era are thrown into considerable turmoil by this event.

The basic reference on menopause in the Cambridge University Medical Library, published in 1976(!), includes an article on "emotional response to the menopause" by Margaret Christie Brown, then a hospital psychotherapist in London, who thought that

> Where overvaluing, undervaluing or imposing of other attributes on the function of reproduction has occurred, difficulty is to be expected with the menopause.

The continuation of her argument involves an unusual twist, which brings her to the point of blaming symptomless women for their lack of symptoms:

> Surveys have shown that the group of women least likely to have menopausal symptoms are single women who have not suffered from dysmenorrhea. The reasons for this must be multifactorial but one important factor is that these women have come to terms gradually over a number of years with non-fulfillment of a female role. It may have been a deliberate way to avoid the vulnerability of being female or it may have been by force of circumstances, in either case she is likely to have faced many of these issues many times and learned to tolerate them over a number of years. So that, rather like living with a seriously ill member of the family, the mourning is done while the patient is alive and often death is welcomed as relief.

Psychiatrists have no option but to blame people for their own suffering; admitting the unhappiness might be justified would undermine the entire rationale of medicating the mind. There can be no suggestion that feeling tired and disillusioned at fifty might be the appropriate response and that convincing yourself that you are happy and fulfilled might be self-deluding to the point of insanity. "Bringing up" children is not necessarily enjoyable; our children are not necessarily nice people and if they are it is not something we can congratulate ourselves upon. In any event, by the time we are fifty our children are likely to be relatively difficult of access. If English and Pearson had actually studied the epidemiology of menopause, they might have observed that women who have most enjoyed mothering often suffer worst at menopause, in which case it is still their fault, because they have been too attached to the mothering role.

Mary Anderson has not the excuse of being a Freudian psychiatrist of the fifties; nevertheless the crisp statement quoted from her book, *The Menopause*, implies that if you have managed your life correctly—if you have a husband and children who all love you, if you have always enjoyed and are still enjoying sex with your husband, if you have a fulfilling job— you are more likely, most likely, perhaps even certain, to whisk through menopause with your usual efficiency. Mrs. Thatcher, according to her goofiest hagiographers, accomplished the climacteric in February 1972; the implication of Anderson's no-nonsense approach is that, if you can't do the same, then you're likely to be a moaning Minnie. If you haven't managed to get a husband, let alone keep him alive and by your side until you are fifty, if you haven't borne any children or have been unable to get the ones you have brought up to treat you decently, if you didn't manage to get a decent education, let alone a decent job, then you'll probably make a hash of the menopause as well. Before dealing with medical treatments for the misery of the climacteric, Mary Anderson permits herself the following non-medical observations:

> Regrettably it is true to say that in all age groups throughout the Western world there is excessive drug use, leading to actual abuse of these drugs. They have become a household by-word—a music-hall (or TV) joke. Who is to blame? The drug firms certainly, the doctor certainly— but patients themselves must take a large share of responsibility. How often do patients go to the doctor's surgery specifically to seek a tablet to calm them down or to buck them up, because they are either anxious or 'stressed' or 'depressed' and feeling low? Modern life itself must take

the main responsibility for all this with its stresses, anxieties and pressures. But do we not create the life we lead, are we not largely responsible for many of the situations in which we find ourselves and should not we be more able to find resources within ourselves to cope rather better without necessarily having recourse to drugs?

While admitting that modern life is not particularly livable, Dr. Anderson chooses to put the words "stressed" and "depressed" in inverted commas; "feeling anxious" is a pretty grudging way of describing an anxiety state. The key to Dr. Anderson's attitude is the question "Do we not create the life we lead?" This is one rhetorical question that should not be answered in the affirmative, for the true answer is, "Probably not, and certainly not if we are women." From the time women first come to consciousness their lives are strenuously molded by others; this conditioning has been so often described at length that there is little point in reiterating it here, but as the point is so central a synopsis may be in order.

From the first weeks of life, when mothers feed boys who vociferate but soothe girls, feed boys more often and longer and praise girls for behavior that they discourage in boys, and when the behavior of fathers may range from total invisibility and distance to sexual abuse, women learn that their fate is not in their own hands. The pattern of responding rather than initiating is early set. If it is not, the chances of a female's life career following Dr. Anderson's ideal are slimmer rather than better. In the co-educational system the girls quickly learn to or decide to let the boys dominate; when sexual activity is initiated it is on the boys' rather than the girls' terms. Though the rhetoric may support equal opportunity, equal opportunity for women in education, professional training and employment does not exist. Women do not understand the systems of self-promotion employed by men; they are not taught the ways in which from their boyhood men establish groups and contacts that will serve them in their professional careers. If women keep up in the professional race, it costs them a great deal more in terms of application and concentration, and yields them a great deal less in terms of human contact. Their male peers, on the other hand, will generally prefer women who do not compete with them.

Nearly a third of Western European women will never marry; the higher a woman's educational qualifications and the better her job, the more likely she is not to marry. Unmarried men cluster at the bottom of the social scale; unmarried women at the top. Married men are the least likely to seek treatment for psychological disturbance; next come single women, next married women. The last, most vulnerable population, selected out of the marriage market, are the single males. Any discussion of menopausal women that assumes that all are or should be married and have had children is based upon a mythical paradigm. Of the women aged fifty or over in Great Britain, nearly half a million will be divorced and never remarried, while more than 3 million will be widows, and three-quarters of a million or more will never have been married; in all, nearly half the total number are single. The largest group of households in Britain are the households with a single occupant. Incidence of divorce increases exponentially, while failure to marry is more and more often refusal to marry, not because the woman is immature or suffers from any other psychological blight, but because the institution of marriage is not designed for women's better health or optimal functioning. More divorces are initiated by wives than by husbands. There are rational grounds for eschewing or ending marriage; the women who choose to do so are taking control of their lives. Survival as a single woman is not easy, but the struggle is one's own struggle. Single women are less likely to form symptoms that demand treatment, simply because they have assumed responsibility for themselves. Even so, menopause doctors see as one of their chief functions the curing of ailing marriages. Despite all the evidence to show that celibates are no madder and often a good deal healthier than the rest of the population, they persist in the irrational belief that regular psychosexual release is essential for the proper functioning of all individuals. . . .

Fortunately for society, if unfortunately for them, women's anger usually expresses itself in self-punishment. Obligingly women internalize resentment which then takes the form of guilt. One of the most interesting results of any test made of the effects of replacement estrogens on personality, most of which were inconclusive, was the conclusion reached by Schiff, Regenstein, Tulchinsky and Ryan in 1979.

Schiff *et al.* included in their assessment three personality scales, the Clyde Mood Adjective Checklist, the Gottschalk-Gleser test and the Minnesota Multiphasic Personality Inventory. These tests assess in all some 26 attributes of personality but in only two of these were any changes observed. Following oestrogen women became less outwardly aggressive but more inwardly hostile. How this is to be interpreted the authors do not say.

Such an observation opens the intriguing possibility that women's submissiveness is mediated by estrogen; deferring to the dominant male is clearly a necessary part of reproductive function. Hens hunker down before the rooster. Receptive she-cats present the nape of the neck to ingratiate themselves with the tom, but unreceptive she-cats turn and fight with as much ferocity as males. It is interesting to consider the famed "mental tonic" effect of HRT as inducing a "contented-cow syndrome." The possibility, ever so faintly adumbrated here, that menopause puts women back in touch with their anger after thirty-five years of censorship by estrogen, is delightful to contemplate. Interestingly, though replacement estrogen facilitates sexual intercourse, it does not restore lost libido, which demands testosterone; in this at least estrogen is clearly the biddability hormone.

It would be foolish to expect the male medical establishment, even when represented by those few female members who care to be associated with menopause, to encourage women to act out their anger or hostility or resentment in middle age. In this best of all possible worlds such feelings are never appropriate. We are only dimly coming to a recognition that the anti-social behavior of demented old women might be an expression of justifiable rage too long stifled and unheard. When we find a frantic old lady in the nursing home cursing foully and soiling herself we are witnessing the end result of long corrosion of the personality. We should not be surprised to find that the most eldritch old hag was once the most self-effacing soul, nor should we assume that her present state has no connection with her earlier condition.

Some of our negative feelings about menopause are the result of our intolerance for the expression of female anger. As little girls and adolescents we feared the anger of our mothers. We sensed that there was a debt of hostility in consequence of all that motherly self-sacrifice and self-effacement, but though we pretend that saying that we had not required either self-sacrifice or self-effacement will stand in lieu of payment, we know better. We are not really surprised when menopausal women spit out bitter home truths to their children, but we pretend that it is the hormonal imbalance that is speaking, turning anger into illness so that we can evade implication in it. Robert A. Wilson embarked on a lifetime career of estrogen prescription because of happenings that predestined his career, principal among them the decline of his "gentle, almost angelic mother":

At the time I could not understand it. What was a boy in his teens to make of a phrase like "change of life"—especially if it was spoken in the tone of voice that in those days was used to mention any number of things then considered unmentionable. How could anything connected with my mother be spoken of in that tone of voice? Yet something terrible was obviously happening. I was appalled at the transformation of the vital, wonderful woman who had been the dynamic focal point of our family into a pain-racked, petulant invalid. I could feel the deep wounds her senseless rages inflicted on my father, myself, and the younger children. It was this frightful experience that later directed my interest as a physician to the problem of menopause.

Poor Mrs. Wilson. If she was as ill as she seems to have been, it must have been particularly dementing to be denied treatment because everyone had a diagnosis—"change of life." She had a teenage child and younger ones; how old could she have been? If she suffered from rheumatoid arthritis or early-onset Alzheimer's and was being tormented with nonsense about climacteric symptoms her rages would have been anything but senseless. Robert A. Wilson based a whole career on amateur diagnoses overheard in his youth. His mental anguish at his mother's rejection of him was exacerbated by another trauma, the sight of a woman's bloated body being torn open by a grappling hook as it was fished from a reservoir near his childhood home. Her suicide too was caused by (whisper, whisper) "change of life." Robert became a crusader. In fact he suffered from an acute form of anophobia (fear of old women).

Anyone who has ever been employed in a business directed by a menopausal woman executive is familiar with another variant of this [menopausal negativity] syndrome. The work week becomes a futile, inefficient round of violent ups and downs, adult tantrums, and pointless chicanery. The woman in a position of authority has a ready-made means of side-stepping the passive kind of menopausal negativism. She is presented with an irresistible and unlimited opportunity to take out her frustrations on her employees.

The middle-aged female employer, dealing with a work force who ignore everything she says because they have decided that she is menopausal, is quite likely to have to think of a number of strategies to get their attention. Criticisms of Margaret Thatcher's way of running her cabinet reflected this mechanism, and doubtless she capitulated to it.

Anophobia is an accretive phenomenon; it causes the kind of treatment of middle-aged women that they react to in a way that seems to justify it. A good deal of the anxiety of the middle-aged woman is caused by her awareness that she is turning into some kind of a harridan, a scold, a jade, a drab, a fishwife, a beldame, but if you can't get attention any other way, what are you to do? There is no way out after all; the vituperative woman, the viper, the virago (vagina dentata) will be told that she has only herself to blame for the negativity that surrounds her. Nagging is painful utterance that the more it is repeated, the more inexorably it is ignored.

Railing has a positive value. Railing in literature, called variously satire, tragic or comic, lampoon, burlesque, invective, has been highly valued, first as entertainment and second as a corrective to abuses, yet though we have female poets we do not have female satiric poets. Though there are hundreds of literary attacks on women by men, there are very few attacks on men by women, and the few we have are almost all answers to unprovoked attacks by men. It is almost as if women's rage is, like women's sexuality, too vast and bottomless to be allowed any expression, for fear it would swamp and capsize the male equivalent. Despite the best efforts of feminists to awaken women's anger and to turn their hostility outward so that it becomes a force for social change rather than the procreator of symptoms, we have failed. With one or two magnificent exceptions, no race of hilarious harridans has appeared upon the earth.

The medicalization of menopause is the last phase in the process of turning all the elements of female personality that do not relate to the adult male into pathology. Virginity is pathology; lack of interest in heterosexual intercourse on demand is pathology; "excessive" involvement in mothering is pathology; middle-aged truculence and recalcitrance are the most pathological of all. Now we have pills for all of them and women are obediently taking them. Doctors cannot change social, cultural, economic or political conditions; they can only try to tailor the patient to fit better into her circumstances. We cannot blame the patient if she asks for help. We cannot blame the doctor if he gives the only help he can. We cannot blame the woman if she experiences the alteration in her responses as an improvement in her health, and chooses to ignore the underlying problems which she cannot solve.

If you are drifting around an empty house that no one wants to spend time in, the children being about their own mysterious affairs and your husband staying late at the office most days, you are oppressed. If you are stagnating in a dead-end job on a miserable rate of pay watching younger people rise past you through the promotion scale, you are oppressed. If you are a widow or a divorced woman struggling to adjust to a new life on your own in one of our unsafe and brutalized cities, you are oppressed. If people take no pains to conceal their lack of interest in you, if people refuse to take you seriously because they have decided that you are menopausal, you are oppressed. If you believe that this state of affairs has been brought about by your inadequacy, and you have to add guilt to your emotional burden, you are not only oppressed, you will feel depressed. You will see yourself as dull, dumpy and gray and not blame the people who do not conceal their lack of interest in you. You are not, after all, interested in yourself.

If you are dumpy and dull and gray, how did you get that way? You might look to your family and your employer and ask as the neglected wife asks in *The Comedy of Errors:*

> *Are my discourses dull? barren my wit?*
> *If voluble and sharp discourse be marr'd,*
> *Unkindness blunts it more than marble hard . . .*
> *What ruins are in me that can be found*
> *By him not ruin'd?*

The evidence seems to show that the more dissatisfied you are with your life the bumpier the ride through the climacteric is going to be, as if your life is trying to jump the tracks. The only people who offer help, the medicos, can offer treatments that will keep you on the rails. The bumps may smooth out but you need to be sure that you want to go on in the same direction. If you do not, there is no reason to feel guilty. If your life has fallen to pieces all around you, there is no reason to feel guilty. If until this point your life has not been under your control, as is all too probable, you can now take control. Indeed, you may have no option. Feelings of vertigo and panic are to be expected, and not to be apologized for. The truth behind the research that failed to find a significant increase in stress at the climacteric is that, though the new life may be more strenuous, it will not be more difficult than the old. Anxiety about aging and worry about health are concomitants of menopausal uproar; when it is over the prospect of illness and decrepitude recedes once more to a manageable distance. Negative feelings are not your fault either. None of it, neither the mood swings, nor the weight gain, nor the loss of interest in sex, nor the insomnia, should incur the added burden of guilt.

Associations en Route to a Bone Scan

Bone . . . bone . . . bone . . . Desertscape
with deadwood, pebbles, scattered femurs,
tibias, with luck a skull, even fossilized.

A Ghanian lady over lunch taught me to eat a chicken
properly: chew the cartilage, crack and split
the bones, suck the marrow, leave splinters.

My shrivelled great aunt was a nurse in World War One:
when all four doctors in the unit died, she performed
amputations in the field. Thanksgivings here, only she

could carve it right. . . . Doctors send small-boned, fair-skinned,
red–haired patients in for imaging. My skeleton, once strong,
designs the shadow of itself on screen. . . . So far I have

consumed myself to 69% of me. . . . Now everywhere I notice bones:
in soup pots, pet stores, butcher shops, battlefields.
At the Smithsonian: tyrannosaurus jawbone, alligator spine,

kneecap of a kangaroo. Snake skeletons strung up like mobiles
rotate, float in bone-dry air. Back home: dog bones, their own,
and those they claim. Will enough of mine be left to chew?

ALMA LUZ VILLANUEVA

Child and Companion

❖

FIRST BLOOD

My daughter calls this morning,
   her voice in wonder:
      "Ashley has her menstrual."

My granddaughter: Yesterday
   I bled old blood, between
     my cycles, to honor

your new blood, the Most Sacred.
   The Goddess in your Body.
   The Goddess in your Womb.

Your mother weeps with happiness.
   Your grandmother smiles with
     joy and nods to sorrow,

child and companion.

To Ashley

Whenever I think of menostop (no, not pause, but stop) now, I think of
my granddaughter, her first menstrual and what that evoked in me, this
poem. She, the child. And companion, her woman's blood. Creativity. Her
power to create. I want her (and all young women) to know this, early on.

43

They have the power. To create: children, books, paintings, cities, science, music, dance, worlds without end. But who will tell her (and all the young, bleeding women)?

It should be us, the older women, the women in menostop, the women (like myself) approaching menostop, the women who have created children, books, paintings, cities, science, music, dance, worlds without end. There aren't many of us (if all the menostop women be counted), but the numbers are definitely growing.

At forty-nine, at the edge of fifty, at the edge of menostop, I pause to look at my beautiful, strong daughter, Antoinette, through her to my beautiful, strong granddaughter, Ashley (who also writes poems), and to myself at eleven when I began to bleed.

It was the year my grandmother, Jesus Villanueva, died that I became a woman. It was Indian summer (close to my twelfth birthday) in San Francisco. It was sunset and I was alone. I decided to climb a building's steel scaffold, though it terrified me to climb alone. Usually I did these daring things with my friend Judy, who was a tomboy like me. Where she was blonde, blue eyed, and had a strong, muscular, boyish body, I had thick, dark, unruly hair (that I kept short or it defied me and became a bush of curls), dark hazel eyes, and a skinny, surprisingly strong body that, in a pinch (as when defending my mother from my abusive stepfather), exploded with what I thought of as "super girl energy."

And so, the sun had set, and the sky rotated above me with bands of pink to red to purple, violet. I knew if I climbed to the top I would see everything so clearly. Like a picture. There might be seagulls in my picture. Or an airplane making a thin trail of cloud. The clouds might form into a familiar face, or into ones that might want to kill me. How did I know? When you're alone anything could happen. What if one of the workmen returned for a wrench, or just to see if some kid was climbing his steel structure? I knew, at eleven years of age, that I was trespassing on masculine territory. Men came here in the daytime, when the sun was out, and created buildings that pierced the sky.

With my friend Judy, I climbed the steel structures. We never complained about the coldness that numbed our hands (we climbed at night), or the heights, as we left the ground. It was nonverbal, never said, but we felt this was how we became boys, like men, and therefore deserved to be in their territory.

As I stood on the exposed earth not yet covered with cement, I looked up to the twelve floors of steel. I knew (in my body) that if I climbed by myself, this picture would be mine. No one else's. If I fell, it would be my fault. If a workman returned and caught me, it would be my fault. If the sky was empty, it would be my fault.

I had to do it. The signal for me was fear. And excitement. That small, dark voice—deep, deep inside me—that persistently said, "I want you to," over and over, until it drowned out all the usual, logical reasons why I shouldn't. Dare.

I began to climb and the steel didn't feel cold like it did later, at night. It still felt warm from the sun. But I had to concentrate: hand to hand, foot to foot, stretching myself higher toward the top, to that faraway sliver of steel that looked unreachable as I stood on the second story beam, alone, and the soft night (the faint smell of steel, oil and men) surrounded me.

Suddenly, I felt unfamiliar, secretive, as though I didn't really care if I died. It was the super girl energy again, but I had nothing to protect or defend. It was just me.

My grandmother, *mi Mamacita*, who had taught me to dream (but never told me, in words, anything about being a woman), had died. My mother was living with her husband, my stepfather, who I hated (I'd knocked him out cold, nearly killing him, when he tried to strangle her). I was living with a woman I barely knew (who I had come to live with by a series of strange circumstances, and who I would come to love in the year that I lived with her). I felt utterly alone in the world, and it seemed as though something waited for me at the top of this incomplete twelve-story building. Its skeleton of steel. So I kept climbing. The words, "I want you to," the command, had become my breath filling my lungs, the blood that pumped my heart (and now, writing this, I remember *mi Mamacita's* words, "*No te dejes!*," which translates, "Don't take any shit!" Or more politely, "Take care of yourself!" She would tell me this, from time to time, when I came in complaining about some mistreatment, and out I'd go to defend myself). Air to lungs, blood to heart, girl to woman.

My mind was empty when I reached the top. The sky was nearly dark. Soon it would be completely dark. The only sound I heard was a steady wind, occasionally a car horn far away on Earth, below. This night, alone, without Judy, I saw the first star appear. Then the others, separate and alone. In school they said the stars were the Hunter, the Lion, things like that. All I saw was each star, alone, bravely shining in the dark, it seemed, for me. They gave me light, each one, separately, and I thought of my grandmother's words, "*El obscuro es la ausencia de la luz. . . .*" ("Darkness is the absence of light.") I wasn't afraid anymore.

Then I felt it. An unfamiliar wetness on my leg, trailing down into my rough, dirty jeans. Quickly, I sat down on the thin steel beam, clutching the scaffolding with my arms and legs. I didn't even think it, *blood*, but I knew. For a long, long time, I sat there absolutely still. I saw myself in the years to come, not as distinct events, but like a blur of feeling—strong, overpowering feeling—as though I were flying through my life wide awake, terrified yet undisturbed. I saw that it was going to be hard, for *her*.

I remember that the stars receded, and that the darkness was complete. I remember that my body was utterly unfamiliar. And so I turned and ran, climbing as fast as I could, trying to touch the ground. But I had seen the picture. My picture. And I thought I had no one to blame but myself.

I was changed. I was different. I was unfamiliar. Now, I was able. To create. Like a woman. My womb had opened up and swallowed me, whole.

This is what happened, but I had no one to translate this experience, this picture (vision) for me (*mi Mamacita*, who raised me, was dead—but she, a full-blood Yanqui Indian from Sonora, Mexico, had taught me to *dream* and to know more than I could say in words). And so I stumbled on without the sustained guidance of older women (it was just your period, the business, the curse, a mess, a taboo mess that stained your clothes and smelled bad, and worse, it was impossible to *be* a boy and trespass on masculine territory, that measure of freedom I'd stolen in my disguise). I stumbled into my teens without a clue to this power. To create. Worlds.

Now approaching fifty, I see I stumbled, fell, and danced occasionally onto the hazardous path of my power. To create. A child at fifteen, seventeen, twenty-one, and finally thirty-six. The poems and stories that came mysteriously at eleven and twelve died out at thirteen, resurfacing with a vengeance at thirty. Poetry and stories in my thirties. My first novel at forty. The endless struggle (and endless joy) to raise my first four creations, each one a novel, each one a world. And my daughter, Antoinette, who I had at fifteen (child and companion), was the mirror to my girl-child, my lost dreams of creativity (she who creates worlds without end), until I reclaimed my lost dreams, firmly and fiercely, in my thirties.

My other children are sons; those privileged by birth, biology and patriarchal culture to have a wider horizon of freedom and privilege. They gave me many years to observe an *unspoiled*, a kind of pure masculinity (which I love and admire, and also recognize in myself as necessary, treasured and hard won).

For example, three years ago I was experiencing a rush of menostop symptoms. I was beginning to feel dire warnings from my body. I was losing some vital strength, some vital energy. I vividly felt my body beginning to cave in on itself. This was at the end of writing two novels and a collection of short stories—a lot of sitting. Though I've always hiked, swam, biked, the *balance* just wasn't right. So, in short, I started a "body program" that included, first, acupuncture, then a take-it-to-the-limit workout and weight lifting program. Three years later, I've lost sixteen pounds, gained muscles where I forgot I had them (coaxing my strength, the energy back). Now I experience the occasional hot flash, but it feels friendly, welcome, and I just let myself sweat, shift gears, let whatever it is, this new energy, do its job—cleanse me. Change me.

As Vicki Noble says in *Shakti Woman** (warning about hormone replacement therapy to avoid hot flashes and menostop symptoms): "Hot flashes happen for a reason, besides the fact that we're toxic and need the release of heat and sweat to relieve the body. *Menopause is preparing us to be healthy old women!* It gives our body a raised temperature during the transition, which probably heals it of potential ills, such as the pervasive cancers that exist in the present moment." Now, coupled with my occasional hot flashes, I also experience my own self-induced sweating/cleansing rituals (of exercise).

I also see that "my warrior" rose up in me, guiding me to that super girl energy that was beginning to become a memory. Who was I at eleven? Where was all that energy coming from, fairly unimpeded? What was all that energy preparing me to do? What if I (and all the other eleven-year-old girls) had lived in a woman-loving, Goddess/God-loving culture? What if there had been (and were *now*) widely accepted rituals for this transition, this huge leap into this crucial phase (girl to woman) of creativity? The challenge of creativity.

These same questions are also for boys (boy to man). Rather than the rituals of drugs, drinking, violence (some media induced version of patriarchal masculinity), the rituals of creativity and challenge, real challenge, like sports, rock climbing, a musical instrument, poetry, stories, a mountain, a mentor, a vision quest *to keep the unspoiled essence* of their masculinity, not encouraged by patriarchal culture. In fact, this essence is under almost constant attack, even as women are (as the girl becoming a woman knows in her bleeding body).

While I was on a walk with my thirteen-year-old son, Jules, he asked me, as we paused to gaze at the ocean: "Is the phallic symbol all the bad stuff like missiles and rifles?" We'd been talking about phallic symbols in our patriarchal culture, and how the media used them for exploitation. I knew, instantly, how crucial this moment was for him, at thirteen, as

* Noble, Vicki, HarperCollins, New York, NY 1991, p. 36.

he approached becoming a man. I said, "Absolutely not. The *real* phallic symbol, the penis, is the symbol of potency and *life*. Like creation, you know?" I saw his face expand, then relax with the sensuality of *knowledge*, and I knew his body, if not his mind, would always remember this moment between us. This answer.

Now, at forty-nine, with my thirteen-year-old son and my twelve-year-old granddaughter in mind, I pause at the edge of menostop, and I see that the bleeding eleven-year-old girl at the top of the steel structure at sunset, in Indian summer, in San Francisco, was androgynous. She was a girl *and* a boy. She was whole, naturally, in a way that I had to learn (step by excruciating step) to become whole again. Always a woman. But androgynous. Whole. Like a child (girl or boy) is whole. This time learned. Earned.

At thirty-five I moved, with my fourteen-year-old son, Marc, to the Sierras and lived in an isolated cabin for four years. A failing second marriage, my grown daughter leaving to live on her own, symbols of the circle that seemed to appear everywhere I looked (seaweed in a circle, a perfectly round stone, a full moon ringed by a circle of light, on and on). Everything seemed to prod me, GO. But where? And then a series of dreams, ending with a clear dream of the cabin, exactly the way it looked.

This dream appeared as a black dot (a dark, tight circle), which I had to pull open, painfully, with both of my hands. First, I had to find my hands in the dream and then, with a great conscious effort—pain running up and own my arms—I instructed my hands not to let go, not for anything. I pulled open the dark, tight circle as wide as I could and saw a cabin surrounded by boulders and trees, with a small meadow in front. The light was strange; not sunlight or moonlight, but dreamlight. It didn't attract me; it compelled me (the words "I want you to" filled my dreaming body). Fear and excitement, dread and curiosity, terror and wonder—my old familiar allies—simultaneously commanded and challenged me ("I want you to"), dared me to do what I felt was impossible at the time. *Where* was this cabin? (I'd never lived in a remote place by myself, and with the responsibility of a teenaged son?) And *why* was I supposed to go there? Because of the circle? Because of the dream?

I found the way, the mountain and the cabin, and I moved, and also found I was pregnant with my third son and fourth and final child, Jules. So I was also going to experience the most primal feminine condition (after deciding, painstakingly, against abortion), with what seemed to be the most primal masculine condition (hermit on the mountain, snow burying cabin, town fifteen miles away, as well as rattlers, mountain lions, bears, coyotes and the local cowboys—that's another story). The absence of the wolf haunted me; they'd killed the last wolf in the area in the forties, I was told. The wolf (one of my dream animals) had guided me there with her sharp nose, eyes and teeth—her strong paws, muscles, her heart.

My first journey up to the Sierras, in *Plumas*—Feathers—County, prompted by a letter from an old friend in Quincy (a former elementary school teacher, she was the only woman wrangler on a guest ranch), was true to the black dot, circle dream. My engine caught on fire. Two men with fire extinguishers, passing me in both directions, jumped out of their trucks (help from the masculine) and put out the fire so quickly my engine suffered only minor damage. I asked myself, Should I continue? After minor repairs, replacing all hoses and burnt parts, I continued.

I had come to that place of transition (as I had on the steel structure twenty-four years ago), that leap into the unknown: creativity. That power. And just as I had as a girl, I felt hunted and unsafe as a woman in the crowded cities of the patriarchal culture (a girl/woman, boy/man, creation/essence-hating culture). I had to do this leap or die. I simply couldn't bear to be a coward. To myself. I simply couldn't bear to give in. To accept my limits. To be a good girl, a "normal" woman (all the time knowing my family, and most of my friends, thought I'd gone too far this time. . . . "And to top it off, she's pregnant, belongs with her husband, for God's sake." I could hear their thoughts).

I desired, at thirty-five, to be *whole* like a bodily need (thirst, hunger, sex), and I knew if I backed away from this inner demand I would die. Perhaps not physically, but most importantly, spiritually. In my soul.

I went looking for my wholeness, looking for the Goddess. I couldn't *see* her in the crowded places where patriarchal time reigned. I couldn't see her, bodily. I had to see her for myself. For my self.

So I stayed on my mountain, in my cabin, and learned to walk at night with "night eyes" over rocks, downed branches, following the sound and curve of a creek (the first few months it was challenge enough to turn off all the lights in the cabin, fall asleep and dream). Then, a year later, I realized walking back to my cabin in the dark by myself: *This darkness, this forest, swallows my cabin, my sons, and me, completely. No wonder I dream these amazing dreams.* (My dreams had become lessons from the Universe, and I the scared-sacred student.) I remember smiling, engulfed by the scent of pine and cedar, and so many night smells I couldn't identify. Yet they all merged into one scent: freedom.

But to make this clear—I didn't wander in naive bliss through the night, the forest, or on my subsequent hikes to the high peaks surrounding my cabin, and later the backpacking trips I took alone to the granite-bowled lakes close by. I either strapped on my buck knife (as I almost always did on my night walks), or packed it in a readily available pouch. There were times I would actually forget to take my knife, and a few times when my shields were tested in dangerous situations (once by a growling mountain lion; another time by two heavily armed—each with guns in holsters and a rifle poking out of his pack—men I met on a lonely trail). Looking back on these incidents, I realize I was meant to "forget" my knife and rely only on my shields (fluidity, intuition, strength, innocence). And the shields held, firmly.

Most important, my stance was to gather as much awareness as possible (like a circle of light, a radar), and tune myself to its continuous message of *what was there*. The forest, the mountains, the night and the day taught me this. They taught me that though I was the hunted, I was also the hunter; and that beyond survival, I was loved and I was the lover. I was loved by the Earth herself. And the Sky. As well as the Cosmos. That I *belonged* in the Cosmos, and that weakness and strength, hatred and love, coward and hero, male and female (the whole) were born in me.

Two months after Jules was born, prematurely, a blizzard blew in that I thought was going to take off the cabin's roof and knock down the walls. My teenager, Marc, was staying the night with a teacher in town; this blizzard stopped all travel. The worst in a century, I read later in the paper. Immense pines and cedars bent to the fierce winds like toothpicks, and the sound of a hundred freight trains roared by my small cabin. I fed Jules every thirty minutes (his preemie schedule), facing simultaneously the fire I kept going all night, and the night outside the windows that merged wind, trees and snow (Sky and Earth) in a perfect and terrifying balance.

Exhausted but alive in the dawn, drinking my first cup of coffee, facing my wide kitchen window, I saw her. The Goddess. The sight was blinding. She was entirely surrounded by cold, cold diamonds: snow. I could see her, *clearly*: high cheekbones, downcast eyes (looking inward), Mayan, utterly serene. Her strength and power flew through my body. I wept with gratitude, relief. Joy. There was no wind at all, absolutely still, but it was freezing out there where she was no more than fifteen feet away. All day I fed Jules within the diamond. All day she stayed with me, utterly perfect. The Goddess.

I had this dream in the Sierras on February 2, New Moon, 1983 (I keep dream journals). I'm shown a basket cradle with chunks of turquoise dangling in a circle, obscuring the contents of the basket cradle. It's the most beautiful thing I've ever seen and I'm overjoyed that it's also mine (although I know it ultimately belongs to the Goddess—and the God). The dream ends:

I have gathered
turquoise for the
cradle of my
power.

It is empty, dark
and full. No human
child sleeps in this,
but the Child of knowledge
and possibility exists
within.

At the edge of menostop, I look at all my *perfect* creations: my thirty-four-year-old daughter, Antoinette, my three sons—Ed, thirty-two, Marc, twenty-eight, and Jules, who's thirteen. I also look at my *im*perfect creations: five books of poetry, three novels, a book of short stories, a new book of short stories, the next novel, the new poems. Then I shut my eyes and I see the basket cradle. It's so beautiful I want to weep and laugh.

I hear the words, "I want you to," but I don't know the exact nature of this command/challenge. I've begun the dreaming (which always translates into living), so I trust this ongoing path of power, my creativity.

I see my fifty-nine-year-old self (thick gray hair, loose to my shoulders), strengthened by exercise and weight lifting, climbing the steel structure. It's Indian summer, close to my sixtieth birthday. It's sunset, and bands of color—pink, red, purple, to violet—wash the sky, changing from moment to moment. I'm terrified, but I'm old enough, and wise enough (at last), to know the twin natures of terror and wonder, how they melt in my mouth, bitter/sweet, and so I simply taste it and sniff the night wind, its many scents that blur into one scent: freedom.

I see *her* (her short dark hair, cut like a boy's). My eleven-year-old self, waiting. There's new, warm blood oozing down her leg, and she's terrified, ashamed, angry. But she's fearless. In her terror, she's absolutely fearless.

She turns to face me. She waits. Child and companion. I feel something on my back, and I know it's the basket cradle. I no longer bleed, so I gather my creations in this mysterious basket, encircled with perfect chunks of turquoise. The turquoise sways in the night wind as I walk toward the bleeding girl. I take her hand (virgin/maiden, virgin/crone) in mine. Her grip is firm. How strong she is. How eager she is to leap. How eager she is for the journey (of her life).

Holding hands, we turn and face the western horizon. We leap. And instead of falling, we fly. The basket cradle is magic (of course), and we have grown feathers/*plumas*.

Together (child and companion), we will create worlds without end. And I know that, though I don't want to die, I'm not afraid of dying ("I want you to").

Menostop is my (further) door, my challenge to accept the mystery of creation. *And I do.*

Epliogue

I wrote this essay before a breast biopsy, after my yearly mammogram revealed a small density in my left breast. I wanted to wait until the biopsy (and the results) were out of the way, but the words "I want you to" compelled me to continue until the last page was written. The night before surgery, just as I began to fall asleep, still awake, I saw (eyes closed) suspended in a black void, two upraised, golden, light-filled hands. They turned, slowly, in the void. I was comforted. They were healing hands. There is a small red line of scar on my left breast (so close to my heart). I don't have cancer.

NORMA FOX MAZER

What's the Big Idea, Anyway?

⁂

Women of my age no longer think of ourselves as on the scrap heap with the advent of menopause, and we're aware that it's not good form to admit that menopause is much more than another moment, another plateau in our lives as women. Still, something has happened: Something profound in our bodies has changed, and that something is impossible to ignore.

When you have menstruated from the age of thirteen to the age of fifty-six, as I did, for forty-three years in other words, the end does not sneak up on you. When it's over, it's over. Gone is your monthly cycle, the miserable lows, the thrilling highs. Gone is the annoyance of inspecting your sheets and underpants to see if they're stained, of getting rid of bloody tampons and napkins. And gone too, is the way in which you count and note the passing of time. When you are menstruating, things happen "just before my period . . . while I was having my period . . . the month I missed my period and was petrified . . ." Gone too, is the possibility that you might produce life again.

I remember my mother remarking once on her relief at menopause: At last, the continual worry about pregnancy was over. But for me it was different. Birth control was a normal part of my life, and to consider having another child also normal. By the time I began menopause, I hadn't had a baby for almost twenty-five years, yet every month I still thought about it. Wondered if it would happen. Hoped it wouldn't. Hoped it would. To get pregnant purposefully or to allow a pregnancy to continue would have been madness, yet it was continually tempting.

Every month, as I bled, in relief and disappointment I remembered that I had a life of my own, work, and four children. Did I really want to continue to populate the world? Did I really want to go back to the nights without sleep? Did I really want the work of caring for a baby, then a toddler, then a teenager? Not really. Yet something in me still yearned. And even at this age, that yearning, that longing, abides in me. Yesterday, on the street, I saw a mother smooth her child's scalp, and instantly I remembered the velvet cap of my babies' heads under my hand and longed for it achingly.

Men, it has been speculated, go through something similar to menopause, but without the drama, without the change marked off abruptly, so there's no ignoring it. One day a man may notice some changes in himself—thinning hair, the penis less elastic and active, but he can choose to ignore it, or pretend to, choose to believe in the myth of the forever potent and attractive male. He can be heartened by novels and movies in which men of sixty, sixty-five, even seventy still make the hearts of young, raunchy women beat hard. Oh, more than that. These women are *panting* to jump into the sack with these older guys, and they do, they do. But who ever heard of a woman of seventy or even sixty making a thirty-year-old man's heart beat hard and his penis rise and thicken in anticipation?

But why am I talking about men, sex, and babies? This was meant to be a meditation on menopause, decay, and death. What a nice triumvirate! What am I saying—have I spilled the beans here? Is this what I really think—that menopause equals decay equals death? *These are the golden years! Age is just a state of mind. You're not getting older, you're getting better.* We all know the slogans. Whole books have been written on the subject of the better menopause, the healthy menopause, and in fact I'm a believer. Keep going, do new things, keep your mind alive and your body active. Good advice, and I do my best to follow it, to carry high the rags and flags of defiance and perseverance.

It's true that these have been good years, in many ways some of the best years. I like to think that I've achieved a certain serenity. I look in the mirror with more dispassion, without the utter despair or the seizing ego of earlier years. After all, the changing of the body happens to everyone. This is what life is all about—you live till you die.

But that's absurd! A truthful absurdity that I'll never understand, not while I have health, family, curiosity, and work. Die? Me? Why? And yet . . . of course I'm getting older, we all are, and at the end is death, which most of us fear, not necessarily in a physical way, but because of its obliteration. So much for serenity and wisdom. So much for truth and philosophy. What is real is that I never minded my monthly bleeding and as it came haltingly, over a few years, to an end, I didn't want to let it go.

I didn't want to give up what it symbolized for me: fecundity, vitality, life giving, my connection to life itself and to all other women, what made me special and apart from men. Nor did I want to give up the thrilling, exultant sexual desire that seized me every month, or even the other side of it, the tears, the days of fumbling and dropping objects, the sudden fits of self pity and depression.

Being there, in those years, in the menstruation nation, was to be vibrant, lush, alive, juicy. And so was I. I was lush, although I didn't know it then. And yet I passed through so much of it as if I were in a dream, the dream of my future, all the things I longed for, and in some ways my body was an encumbrance, something I thought about too much and which drew for me too much attention. I was accustomed to men looking at me, I was often made nervous by it although there wasn't a street I could step on, a room I could step into, a man I could be near without my skin leaping in desire and response.

Now men don't look at me much anymore. No more their swift, tense, admiring glances. All about are girls and women with thick, beautiful legs, wonderful hair, smooth skin. So that's gone, and I miss it. And something else I miss—that ravaging, aching, coveting, craving walk through the world in which every man I saw drew the thought, *Yes, you . . . no, not you . . .* Desire is there still, but so subdued!

A friend says about her encroaching menopause, "No, I don't want this! It's unfair! What's the big idea, anyway?"

Maybe the big idea is that as women we live in a reality we can never escape. We bleed every month for decades, and then we don't. The bleeding reminds us continually that we are tied to life in a way that males are not, and the end of the bleeding is a reminder that our bodies are changing, aging, following the inevitable, irresistible, irreversible law of all life. The cessation of bleeding tells us as nothing else does that the illusions of youth—of eternal youthfulness, of enduring vitality, of resurrection each morning, of attractiveness undiminished—are only that. And that the end of life—of our own precious life—is quite suddenly, if not overpoweringly, close; at least, at last, in sight. We begin counting.

In my early years, I entered the world like a new swimmer in a vast ocean. Sometimes I seemed in danger of drowning, sometimes the waters parted before me. I flailed away, swimming in my own ocean of lust, inhibition, shyness, and eager self-consciousness. My face flamed at attention, I wanted to vanish into corners and stare at others, listen to their conversation, and pluck them out of life and into my stories. Looking at old pictures of myself, I'm astonished at the glowing beauty I see there. She's someone I was never comfortable with. I knew I was "pretty," but now I see the skin, the hair, the eyes—I took all for granted, even lightly scorned these gifts of nature because I hadn't earned them.

I no longer flail at the world in the same way. I am on comfortable terms at last with myself. I like meeting men as people and not as possible sexual partners. There is, after all, something to be said about coming to this point in life.

And yet, and yet . . . I go in circles. Is it ever possible to escape the regret? More times than I care to remember I think of the famous dictum: Youth is wasted on the young. Indeed, indeed, indeed. At least, on the young me. The years during which I menstruated were years of rushing down what seemed an endless road into my life, years of vitality, energy, and a sense of timelessness, the time when I always had time ahead of me, when everything still remained possible. Menopause was a sharp turn in the road. I still go forward, but the idea that the road will come to an end is no longer unthinkable.

SARA McAULAY

(In)Visibility

✠

Even during the years when I was straight, married, actively engaged in childbearing and child-rearing, I never defined myself in terms of my reproductive capabilities. So I was surprised to find, when I started skipping periods, that the prospect of entering menopause depressed and frightened me. In part it was the horror stories I'd heard all my life. I'd have hot flashes. I'd have night sweats and mood swings; I'd become what the men in my ex-husband's family called a "Menopause Minnie"—shrill and irrational, sexless, unattractive. My cunt would dry up. I'd grow a beard. And I figured that the very existence of those worries was proof my fate was sealed, because such fears were themselves pretty irrational *(it's starting already!),* and I could get pretty shrill, at least in my own mind, when I thought about what was in store for me.

To whatever degree these things are genetically linked, there was nothing to suggest that I'd have a particularly difficult time. My mother hadn't had flashes. Nor was she any more moody or irrational than she had a right to be, given her circumstances at the time her periods ceased. So what if in later years she occasionally tweezed a hair or three from her chin? That was hardly what you'd call a beard. What was I worried about?

All my life I've been blessed (knock wood!) with an efficient and trouble-free body that did what it was designed to do without my having to give it much thought or anything more than routine maintenance. I still have my tonsils and my appendix; my plumbing always hummed along as smoothly as the rest. I never had cramps. I got pregnant quite literally without trying, had an uneventful pregnancy and normal delivery. I nursed my son, to his satisfaction and my own.

57

Why should menopause be any different?

For years I didn't know. But I knew that it was. I'd wake in the night and lie staring out my window at the branches, black on gray then black on rose in that last half hour before my alarm when off, and I'd wonder just what the hell my problem was.

Getting older? *Memento mori?* First you get bifocals, then you hit menopause, and then you get shrill and irrational and you grow a beard and quit having sex and then you get old and die? Something like that?

*Some*thing like that. Of course I had the bifocals already, and they made me queasy, and of course I wasn't thrilled with *get old and die.* But I didn't look forty-nine; I didn't feel forty-nine. I had an active sex life and a chin that didn't need shaving. I was still trying to decide what to be when I grew up. Pushing fifty had its drawbacks, maybe (minor injuries seemed to take their sweet time healing, for example), but nothing to lose sleep over.

Ah, but that was *pushing* fifty. What would happen when the big five-o pushed back? Would this be when whatever it was that was going to dry up, did so—dried up and blew away?

This wasn't something I could have asked my mother about, even assuming she hadn't died years earlier. I couldn't have asked her, or any of my aunts or female cousins either. To hear most of them tell (or not tell) it, they'd never *had* sex, at least not in living memory. Vaginal discomfort? To hear them tell (or not tell) it, none of them owned a vagina of any description, let alone one in which dryness might qualify as a change worth remarking. I figured I was scared and depressed at the prospect of the possible loss of my sexual appetite, or of reduced responsiveness, or of being seen as less attractive and desirable. I was scared and depressed at the prospect of stepping over the line separating bifocal-dependent but active middle age from that nice euphemism, "older" (meaning, one-foot-in-the-grave-and-the-other-on-a-banana-peel).

All of the above strike me now as perfectly reasonable fears, given the youth-loving, sex-fixated culture we live in. Lose your youth, lose your looks; lose your looks, lose your sexuality; lose your sexuality, disappear. Those messages are out there, ubiquitous, in the air we breathe; in our toothpaste and blue jeans and cars, in whatever the marketplace offers. Smarter and more independent-minded women than I have bought into them—even, in some cases, as they swore that they had not.

It's taken me a while to understand that my worries weren't about sexuality and attractiveness, particularly, or even exactly about aging. They were about being a fifty-something woman in a society that still judges females by criteria quite different from those it uses for males. And while said society might have finally evolved to the point that some women over forty can play political and economic hardball with the guys, and a few retain their aura of erotic possibility into their fifties and well beyond, generally speaking, the "older" woman who isn't a highly paid, highly visible professional is damn near invisible.

I didn't want to be invisible, any more than I wanted to be a joke, a Menopause Minnie.

I was afraid of the loss of color and energy of all kinds; the leaching away of wildness and juice and noise and smoke and the ability to travel light and the willingness to do so at a moment's notice. I was afraid not so much of growing old or dying as of growing timid and tame.

My first indication that, yes, the dread *it* was finally happening came on a ten-day backpacking trip. I'd figured my period would start before I got home, and brought along what should have been a generous supply of tampons. Sure enough, three days out, it started. No problem. Two days passed, then three; no problem except the bleeding seemed heavier than usual. Four days, then five, and a heavy, clotted flow with no sign of abating. I was a) out of tampons, and b) beginning to panic because my periods never lasted more than four days, but this one seemed to have settled in for the duration. And there I was, in the northern Pennsylvania wilds, wadding up toilet paper from my quickly dwindling supply, rinsing my underpants five or six times a day, feeling weak and sick and wondering if I had cancer, growing surer by the hour that I did, and if not cancer something else, nearly as dire. I couldn't bring myself to face the fact that at my age, while I might actually have some pathological condition, there was a likelier explanation for what turned out to be a two-week-long near hemorrhage.

My mother's menopause was brought on artificially, by radiation treatment for persistent hemorrhaging that was possibly menopause related (she was in her mid-forties), exacerbated by stress. My father was dying of leukemia, and she really had no one to turn to. This was in the early fifties. No support groups; the church said accept the will of God. Psychotherapy was for crazy people, and cathartic shows of emotion were for the weak, for those who were "not our kind." In our family, whatever your problem was, you toughed it out and chalked up cosmic brownie points, redeemable in heaven. No wonder Mom's system rebelled.

I've been thinking about my mother a lot recently; she comes into my mind at unexpected times, bearing unexpected gifts, admonitions, accusations. Just as I was drafting this piece, for example, I recalled an incident that had lain dormant for almost forty-five years.

I remember a train, going somewhere, probably from Alexandria to Roanoke, where we had kin, or Richmond, where my brother was in school. My father was still alive, but doesn't figure in this memory, which is graphic and intense and connected to no context except the train. I am maybe nine. I accompany my mother to the restroom, which is a typical train restroom, tiny and cramped. Nevertheless, we both go in. I pee and then my mother does, or in the memory I think that's what she's doing. But maybe not. The flow keeps on and keeps on coming, and it doesn't smell like urine, exactly. It smells familiar, but not like anything I can name. It keeps on, keeps on, while I pretend not to watch, pretend not to be fascinated, and a little bit splashes on the toilet seat and it's not pee at all, but blood. My mother changes her Kotex; she says something wry, like "what a nuisance" (as strong a statement as she was likely to allow herself), then wrings out and rolls up the soaked pad and wraps it in paper toweling, which turns a sudden shocking red. "What a nuisance." She washes her gory hands. Her face is pale and sweating. We return to our seats without another word.

Looking back, it's hard for me to believe that this happened; hard to believe that my mother, squeamish as she was about most bodily functions, would take me with her into the cramped and intimate space of a train restroom while she changed her sanitary pad at all, let alone when things were as out of whack as they obviously were. I ask myself if it's possible I dreamed this, or made it up—I *do* make things up, it's true. But not this time.

I thought, that day in the train, that my mother was dying; that she would bleed to death and it would be my fault because I did nothing to help her. But she didn't ask for my help, or tell me what she needed. I was supposed to know what she needed, and how to give it to her. Alone in the Pennsylvania night, rinsing and wringing out the T-shirt I used when the last of my toilet paper was gone, I might have remembered that incident and seen some connection, but I did not. I rinsed and wrung out my soaked shirt and hoped I wasn't dying, hoped that whatever I had was something western medicine could cure.

It's been almost a year now since . . . what do we call it, Punto Final? The Last Hurrah? Plenty of time for whatever endocrine driven uproar was going to make its dry, hot, hairy presence known to do so. Nothing. Okay, an occasional, shall we say, *warm* flash. Better than ever sex, boundless energy and high spirits. Should I feel left out? I don't.

What I feel is a mix of relief and amazement, frustration and anger. Relief because apparently I am to be spared most of the discomfort experienced by some. Amazement bordering on awe when I step back from myself and acknowledge the path our bodies follow. But I'm frustrated because, despite my history of rollicking good health, I'm statistically at high risk for both breast cancer and osteoporosis—and the hormone replacement therapy indicated for one is contraindicated for the other. It makes me angry that no one can give me advice that feels like anything other than guesswork. Estrogen alone? Estrogen and progesterone? Herbal remedies? Herbal and hormone? No intervention? Snake oil? Good thoughts? It's a crapshoot; the studies contradict each other and doctors disagree.

Menopause and related conditions, including breast and uterine cancer and osteoporosis, have recently emerged as hot topics. Books. Talk shows. Major articles in major magazines. Good, I say; it's about time. But I worry that interest will quickly peak and just as quickly wane. I worry that our national attention span has already been stretched thin over this topic. Maybe tomorrow I'll wake up to an All New! Improved! Hot! Sexy! Condition/Pathology/Ethical Issue du Jour, and the compelling concerns of women my age will be out there on the remainder stack with anorexia and surrogate moms and the rest of yesterday's news. Out of sight and out of mind.

Invisible, in other words. I don't want that to happen. Don't plan on letting it happen. Not to me, and not to other women my age either, if I can help it. I'm opting for visibility: We are here. Visibility: We have lives—complex and interesting lives. Visibility: We are women. This has not changed.

Here is a story to end with.

Once upon a time there were two women. One was fifty, one was fifty-five when they met and fell in love. Anyone who noticed might have told them they were too old to be that passionate—it was embarrassing to think about, even for them. All that necking in the car! Like kids! Phone calls at midnight and at five A.M. The little poems and notes and pictures shoved under office doors (I forgot to mention that they worked in the same building) at *great risk of discovery*, which was half the fun, of course. But no one noticed. They were too old to be interesting.

Once in a while the women went dancing. They went dancing at straight clubs!

And because they were *old*, no one paid much attention. In a way that was nice. Before they were living together, when they were just having an affair and weren't sure they wanted the whole world to know about it, it was very nice. Protective coloration. They could walk arm in arm on the street and it was just *two older women walking*; two women whose combined ages, as they like to remind each other, added up to more than a hundred years. No one looked twice at them. They could hold hands as they strolled through the park. *Two old broads*, who cares? Once or twice, feeling pretty bold, they even kissed in public. On the lips! In broad daylight! People smiled at them: *such good friends!*

After a while, though, after they were living together, still passionate, still leaving each other silly little romantic surprises under the office door but feeling like a couple and wanting people to recognize that about them—after a while it began to royally piss them off that people dismissed them that way.

How dare they? the women asked each other. How dare they deny us the very essence of what we feel? How dare they look at us and see just friends, roommates not lovers; how dare they assume we don't *do* it? Two *older women*, one quite gray, *getting it on*. We do!

Unthinkable!

They tried to think what to do. And it seemed to them that their lives were filled with color and energy of all kinds. They felt wild and, yes, juicy, and they made all kinds of noise. They could be out the door and on the road on ten minutes' notice, on their way to adventure. It was hard to believe that no one noticed; no one so much as blinked. Shouldn't the whole world be cheering them on?

First they had to get the world's attention, but this had been their problem all along. Clearly, they were going to have to go for the outrageous, though outrageous really wasn't their style. What to do, what to do? They didn't quite have the nerve to strip naked and make love on the lawn in front of city hall at high noon, though the idea had its appeal. Something that crazy, that noisy and wild. Something no one could ignore. They thought and thought, eyeing the city hall lawn with its sparkling fountain and its pigeons and noontime strollers. Lots of noontime strollers. "Maybe if we were younger," one of the women began.

"Maybe when we're older," said the other.

They looked at each other and laughed.

ELLEN GILCHRIST

The Wine Dark Sea

☒

I'm sick of everyone else having all the fun talking about menopause. I want to get my oar in. I went through menopause. My experience is just as good as anyone else's. Here's what happens. You stop menstruating. Blood stops running out of your body six days a month. You stop ruining all your silk underpants. You stop having to borrow Tampax from strangers in public restrooms during ball games and ballets and movies. (The first one I borrowed was at a movie theatre in Harrisburg, Illinois. I was thirteen and it was a Kotex since Tampax hadn't been invented yet.)

Sometimes you can't borrow one. Sometimes you have to stuff your underpants full of Kleenex or your handkerchief or a sock. Then you slink home full of shame.

Back to the menopause. First you don't menstruate every month. You menstruate some months and not others. This is okay except that you think you're pregnant all the time. I made a lot of money off that experience by writing a book about a woman who has a baby when she is forty-four. It is called *The Annunciation* and has sold about three hundred thousand copies in the last twelve years.

The other thing that happens is that you have hot flashes. This is very exciting if you let it be. You are walking across a room minding your own business and suddenly you are consumed by heat. Your body heats up to about a hundred and four. This happens in seconds. You break out in a sweat. Then the heat passes and only the sweat remains. You have been reminded of mortality and death and where you are in space and time. You are in the universe of process and decay, of atoms and particles and human biology, that frail and delicate phenomenon to end all phenomena.

Take that excitement into your soul. Understand who and where and what you are. You are awake now, not in the stupor in which most of us live our lives. Rilke said it is as though our life is a room but as we grow older we only inhabit a small part of the room, pacing up and down before a window, tracing and retracing our steps. He said, "We must accept our experience as vastly as we possibly can; everything, even the unprecedented, must be possible within it."

Of course, for this you need courage and the strength to be alone with your own mortality. You have to forget what the outside world thinks of you. You have to push aside the trashy notions of our culture. You have to remember mountains and rivers and the motions of planets. You have to remember snow and steam and your life in the womb. You have to bend down to your own unimaginable curiosity, to the dazzling impossibility of being here, in this form, on this earth, with this day before you to be lived. You have to grow up.

There is always a lot of free-floating anxiety in any psyche and it will latch on to anything it can. Menopause has always been fertile ground for anxiety. Don't give in to this syndrome.

Take estrogen if you can. Or don't take it. Exercise at least an hour a day. Hard, intense exercise, long walks or bicycles rides, aerobics or dance classes. Make exercise a priority. Use it as a shield against fear. Eat intelligently, drink bottled water, take vitamins. Sit in meditation, listen to music, turn off the television set. Don't be afraid. The best is yet to come. These are the high passes where the air gets thin and the light becomes translucent.

"Keep warm, old man," the boy said. "Remember we are in September."

"The month when the big fish come," the old man said. "Anyone can be a fisherman in May."

MONIFA A. LOVE

First to Last

⌗

1.

Among the water lilies, slithery pads and roots,
    in Styrofoam water wings, flowered cap
and turquoise suit, I am inflated like the sky,
    swollen with the pride of almost swimming.
My great aunt is in the water, her left hand a visor,
    her right towing me ashore. She is scraping
leeches from my body. There are tiny red dots
    along my arms and legs. She rubs my skin
with yellow juice and makes me drink. "Stop jumpin',
    they're off. Now your blood'll smell of marigolds."

Cross-legged on the floor examining small red drops
    I don't hear Aunt Jessie pulling up the stairs,
padding across the open room we share. Crumpling
    the evidence in my lap too late, "That's good," she says,
"between field work and babies I never knew."
    "Never knew?" "Anything. Who. When.
If someone was coming or gettin' ready to go."
    She pins folded white linen fragrant with cedar,
rose and long-held keepsakes. I'm bulky between the legs
    like a boy. I keep looking down. "I've a mind for pokeno."

The shiny red chips are railroad lights, strawberry
    gelatin, devil eyes and secret codes. They are Harlem

65

streets, sparkling clothes, my aunt's dreams of applause,
        unafraid men and a life away from tobacco, Florence,
South Carolina, and the seesaw of light skin. Rising
        slowly from the table, "Don't mess with the cards,"
her hips and shoulders move like she's a lemon meringue woman,
        satiny crowned and toothsome, her voice
like scuppernongs, "Not a soul to ease the pain, you bleed
        in vain, you've got the bleeding hearted blues."

2.

I dream of my ex-husband
his red clover kisses pungent
and disarming   medicine
his skin warm sand
powder soft   consoling
my outlet to the sea
his fragrant fall into my body
wisteria
I enjoy this foreign man
whose face I think I know
"come with me, be with me
it's not too late"
        "who are you?"
I watch his hand move to his heart
rise and fall with his chest
"who you believe"
    My brittle answer is a long, slow breath
    my heavy head turning side to side
    I feel my blood in my throat
    spilling over
    a beet red line trickles out the corner
    of my mouth down my breast into my navel
    and disappears
    it follows the path of our woundings
    sirens   crimson lights   white rooms   curtains drawn
    to a baby who drinks our descent
    and slips away
"please?"

3.

My aunts and female cousins have no wombs.
Gone.
Mother gone.
Grandmothers gone.
Aunt Jessie long gone.
Who will say she felt fallow
voided
unchained
excused
capricious
jubilant?
Who will tell me she felt nothing
everything
the same?
Who will nod if I can speak
of babies lost
doors closed
regret?
Who will laugh at me
when I whisper
about escape
and breathe hard?

S. HOLLY STOCKING

Mirror Dancing

On the drive to her ballet class, my thirteen-year-old daughter studies her reflection in the passenger side mirror. She turns first one way, then the other, smiling now with lips parted, now with lips closed, flicking her hair away from her face. Then she laughs, a high breathy little laugh and checks for the effect. At a stoplight, face forward, and moving only my eyes, I peek at this display, and stifle the muscles that want to smile. My daughter is pressing her left index finger to the tip of her nose, and she is lifting it ever so slightly. . . .

I had forgotten what it was like to preen like a bird, to pirouette close to a mirror then gingerly edge back, turning from side to side, tilting chin up then down, like a cockatoo in a cage, waiting to be fed. But in the last year, it has all rushed back. I call it mirror dancing, and it is not only my daughter who is engaging in it these days. With growing frequency, I find myself eyeing my face sideways in the bathroom mirror, studying the skin that has grown slack under my chin. If I pinch the skin between thumb and forefinger, it forms a ridge that flattens gracefully, like oven-heated cookie dough. It does not snap back the way it used to, the way my daughter's cheeks do when she pinches them to red. I sigh and look straight on in the mirror, pressing my fingertips toward my ears at the outer edges of my cheeks, pulling taut the skin that has begun to sag into jowls. . . .

Like many mother-daughter pairs of our generations, my daughter and I have arrived at the cusps of the menstrual cycle together. Books on "the change" have prepared me for the physical and emotional changes I am experiencing, and a sex education class has prepared my daughter for the monthly cycles that will be hers for much of the rest of her life. But nothing has prepared either of us for arriving at these changes at precisely the same time.

Nothing perhaps, except her infancy. When my daughter was a newborn, I sometimes confused us, one with the other: I would see a pimple forming on her chin, and I would scrub a mole on mine. I would spy a fleck of oatmeal on her forehead and attempt to pluck it from my own. Her face would redden with the heat, and I would find myself shedding layers of my own clothes. There are moments now when similar confusion overtakes me: My daughter's face breaks into zits, mine into pores. Her body puffs out; mine blimps out. Enraged by some small slight, she slams her bedroom door; in tears, I feel the urge to slam mine, too. There are days when we both want to crawl into holes.

And yet there are the obvious differences: My daughter's dance is choreographed by rapidly dividing cells and by hormones released to swirl her into womanhood, to give her the scent of a desirable female, to sever the invisible cord that has tied her to me since she arrived squalling and needing in a bath of blood. My own dance is choreographed by hormones and cells winding down, tiring in the years that once would have been called old age. The blood that my body shed each month since my own twelfth year has sputtered to a stop. And as my daughter readies to release her own blood, I prepare with mixed feelings to turn over the unused napkins on the shelf in my bedroom closet. My daughter can't grow up fast enough; I grow old too quickly.

In three years my daughter will be driving. Two years after that, she will graduate from high school. At thirteen, she is already thinking of college. She is impatient with the present. She wants to be treated as an adult. But less as an adult member of the family than as an adult stranger who moves in, fails to pay the rent, shows up for dinner, and complains that there's nothing decent to eat in the house (or on her plate). When I ask her how was school, she thinks I'm being nosy. When I ask if she would like to go shopping, she looks at me like I'm certifiable; she would like new clothes, yes, but she does not want to shop with her mother, she tells me. "No one shops with her mother anymore! No one." When I drop her off at the movie theater at the mall, I wait to be sure her friends arrive. She is mortified, even after they fail to show. "When you're thirteen, mothers don't wait around!" she lectures. "And why are you carrying that coffee cup into the mall?! Nobody walks around with a coffee cup in the mall! And why do you have to wear those combs in your hair?"

Suddenly, I am old and frumpy and stupid. I am my own mother—the woman I was convinced at my daughter's age I did not want to be seen with, ever. She talked and laughed too loudly. She yelled at me for no apparent reason, she was a hypocrite, and her taste in clothes—and boys and just about everything else—was horrible. I was sure she could not bear the differences between us, and long after adolescence I rejected her because it was the only way I knew to become myself.

I ought to be able to slough off this latest mother-daughter confusion. The mother I once rejected is nearly eighty; her body is frail; she has cataracts, high blood pressure, and osteoporosis. Still, she manages a home, travels, sends me a book about "the change," and tries not to complain about her rapidly failing health. I see her now as the strong, courageous woman she must have always been—flawed as a mother, yes, but the best mother that she was prepared to be. In my saner moments, I know my daughter will someday see her own mother with kinder eyes. But in less sane times, when I am flushed with years and my daughter is mortified by my very being, I am apt to forget all this and take her current feelings—my own feelings at her age—as fixed for the rest of my days.

It is at such moments that I must struggle for wisdom, for all the measured thoughts that I have acquired, along with the sags, the wrinkles, and the rounder lines. It sometimes helps, at moments such as these, to remind myself of the lessons that the weight of experience impresses: I am separate, I am whole, and beneath these creaking ribs, love beats and the spirit flies.

It can help, too, to notice beneath the rebelliousness of adolescence, the strengths that are my daughter's. Even now, before experience has grabbed her by the throat, my daughter knows things it has taken me half a lifetime to learn: She appreciates that people have differences. She accepts that she and her friends are not perfect. She appears to know that she is loved.

Several years ago, a friend gave me a poster. It was a reminder to women that we don't need to become our mothers. At the time, I passed it along to my daughter. Thinking of my own mother recently, thinking of her dimming eyes and the painful crack in her back, I remembered the poster. Not long after, I asked my daughter if I could look at it, but she had thrown it away. She explained that she hadn't thought she would need it; it had never occurred to her to worry that she might become like me.

More recently, as I drove the two of us to the bookstore, my daughter tried to explain yet again why she no longer wants me to accompany her places. Except for repeating again and again, "It's just embarrassing!" she was singularly inarticulate. I sighed and cut to the bottom line. "It's just that I sometimes wish we were closer," I said. My voice was full of gravel.

My daughter looked over at me then, and reached from the passenger side of the car to pat me on the shoulder. "We're closer than you think," she said softly. And then, as quickly as a hummingbird, the moment was gone.

My daughter is a dancer. Except for mirror dancing, I am not. But sometimes, in my wiser, more contented moments, I imagine us dancing together. The last time I did this, I imagined a beautifully choreographed ballet set against a backdrop of full-length mirrors. My daughter and her friends were in brilliant red feathers, *en pointe*, my friends and I feathered in shades of grays, in canvas slippers.

I imagined that my friends and I encircled our daughters, moving close, then back, fanning their bright plumes. Suddenly, one of the young dancers broke free and led her friends in perfectly synchronized leaps to the back of the stage. There, they paused before mirrors, cocking their heads first one way, then the next, raising their arm-wings and studying the effect. We mothers approached the mirrors ourselves then, studying our daughters' images and our own. We flapped our wings to catch our daughters' attention, but they acted as if we weren't there. We flapped again, but they had eyes for no one but themselves. Finally, weary from all the looking, we tired and swooped off the stage.

Within moments, one of the younger dancers backed off from the mirror and stopped. At her feet lay a faded feather. Spying it, she looked around, as if searching. . . . Finding no one, she paused, gingerly picked up the feather at her feet, and clasped it to her breast. It was my daughter. My heart, or maybe it was just the feather, I can't be sure . . . it fluttered.

JANET BURROWAY

Changes

❖

HAIR

I was maybe thirty-five, six. I was in a high bed between enameled walls for one of those operations that needn't be named because it's unspellable. The black nurse arrived with basin, towel, soap, razor, and ready cheer. I moaned, and the muscles of my stomach clenched, maybe with fear, maybe with more minor dreads, remembering the shaving of my pubes when my first son was born, my angry certainty that it was unnecessary—that anger silenced by my ignorance—and the long scratchiness of the hair growing out.

Now the buoyant nurse told me to turn on my side and raise a knee. Oh, I said, relieved, she wasn't going to shave me then?

"Just in back! Oh, lord, love, I'm not going to take your glory!"

She drew the vowel out, voluptuous. I sighed with relief and pride. My gloory. It was so. The hair on my head is fine and straight, the stuff I shave under arms, on shins, is negligible and spiky. But there! Then! A nether Afro, black with red highlights, luxuriant, an ebullient mass. Brushed, it would spring back instantly into ringlets. The American euphemism "beaver" is ignorant, a thick flat metaphor, nothing like. But a "bush," yes, resilient, silky, and sunny; it was a ready growth, warm May sprout, moss and glossy.

I remember the delicate baldness of girlhood, and how as a child I a little fearfully imagined myself in that goatee. Now, the other side of glory, I look at the thinness of my fur and find it somewhat stingy of nature, mean-natured, not necessary, that I have become thus sparse.

Nobody, I take it, minds but me. It is not a death, a serious separation, is not grief. I seem to function better, come to that, than in the glory days.

Hormones are keeping my bone marrow dense, knowing better how to choose a lover keeps me at better joy.

More. I'm lucky. By the time she was my age my grandmother wore on her head a half-wig called a transformation; by this age my mother's skull showed blue-white beneath the "poodle" cut crimped to hide it; in his forties my brother was egg-pated above his beard. I've escaped this Pierce-side-of-the-family tendency to baldness, and my barber who styles himself a stylist tells me that there's no sign I'm thinning on top.

Only below, this bush of best youth, this kinky growth, this sable V, this little lawn, this springing grass, this private isle, reminds me that the very hairs are numbered.

What do you say to the losses of age? Oh, well. Oh, well.

TONE

K., who has a younger lover, moans that he's always wanting her on top. Why does she dislike this? I thought we fought through the fifties, the sixties, to gain the right to that position. I thought we wanted access to men who allowed, liked, preferred, requested it. I thought it was a distinct advantage of the younger lover, the liberated generation. I thought we fought to overturn "missionary" laws.

No. I know perfectly well what she means. She says, "Your face is so much better on your back."

This is not very articulate, but it brings that discovery back with a rush. I was doing something sweet. P. had no bedroom mirror and I had a spare. This one was big and clear and old, with a many-times white-painted frame of heavy Victorian gingerbread. The glass was loose in the frame and I was going to secure it before taking it to him for long-term loan—an indefinite, commitment sort of loan. I drove the little nails around the back of the frame, covered the join with heavy tape, then turned it over on the carpet to check the paint for nicks. Straddled hands and knees over the silvered glass I caught sight of my face. Stopped shocked. I watched the crawling creature warily. Its skin and chin pulled forward off the bone, the jowls slid into the hollow of its cheeks. The bold eyes hid under the shelf of brow, which furrowed with the grainy pucker of the pull of center earth. The quality of the skin was that it foreshadowed its disintegration into cells of infinitesimal size. The opposite of taut is not, apparently, loose, but netlike. The wrinkles I am accustomed to seeing in my face are few and deep—laugh lines, crow's feet, furrows. These were hairline fissures dividing cell and cell.

This was not me. I know my bad side from my good, I know I am capable of posturing for the mirror, I know what I look like without makeup, I have even imagined my own skull. But this was not me, not me. I hung over gravity, I regarded myself gravely: I became grave.

Crepe is death's fabric.

All epidermis aspires to the condition of elbow.

Aging is nature's own *verfremdungseffekt*.

Because the idea of "tone" is a metaphor from music, I have co-opted the word "semiquaver" to describe this quality of skin. Dutifully doing the morning exercises that keep my spine from hurting, legs straight over my torso I watch my knees fall toward me, microcosms of erosion, miniatures of buckling earth, tan temblors of the meaning of change. The flesh semiquavers on my knees. I have become rather fond of the sight.

I ran into a very young woman at the vet's. In other times I'd have called her a girl. Her legs were thin and without definition but with adequate fullness of lovely flesh. Her ankles ran straight from her calves into her socks and sneakers. Her skin was flawless Florida tan, butterscotch-pudding smooth. I admired this skin for several seconds before I realized that I did not envy and did not *want* it. I would call its texture callow. A lovely accident of flesh, and lo, I'll choose my own.

You think I'm lying for rhetoric's sake, but don't underestimate the part of change that happens behind the skin. The beauty of bark, or woodgrain; the sound of "texture": text-sure. I finger my lover's elbows forgivingly. We embrace in the frame of gingerbread. I like his aging. I believe, know, that he likes my flesh buckling, semiquavering, text-sure. I like us liking our aging. We feel, to me, to have traded some quality of mere appearance for superior sight.

I climb on top.

HILL

Aunt J.J., eighty-two, is touring Alaska once again with W., her companion of forty years. W. is the elder but will not say by how much. I keep their itinerary on my calendar because by the time I get back from England they will be packing for Switzerland, and we'll need to catch up. After Switzerland it's the Delta Gamma convention, and then the World Future Conference. They live, when they're at home, in the Ozarks of Branson, MO, and J.J. has lately taken to country western. W. keeps up a correspondence with some hundred and twenty people they've run into on their travels. Mornings they power walk, though they just call it walking. "It's lucky," W. says, "once you have the time, to have the health, the means, and the inclination still to travel."

Meanwhile I talk to my stepmother, G., also eighty-two, in the nursing home in Arizona. First I call the nurse, who wheels G. to her own phone; then I call her phone, which the nurse puts in her hand. G. can walk, but won't; so the circulation has dwindled, and her legs are purple blue. Amputation has been mentioned, though not to her. As soon as she hears my voice she begins to cry. "I just don't know how to cope with these interviews anymore," she says.

"What interview is that, dear?"

"Oh, well, you know your dad is always being interviewed by these magazines, and you never know exactly how much you ought to tell them."

My dad died in 1987. So far as I know he was never interviewed by a magazine. G. straightens the sob out of her voice and sighs. "It seems like I just can't figure it all out. I don't know how to keep everything together."

She knows, and means, that her mind is going, almost gone—though she articulates very clearly what she wants. She wishes she could dig a long ditch and just lie down in it and not get up. She wishes an angel would come and lift her out of all this mess.

I ask stupidly if she got the book, the sweaters. Does she see the picture of me and P. on her dresser? Does she remember that we came out to visit her a few weeks ago?

"Couldn't you come over just for a few minutes now?"

"I'm in Florida, though. It's two thousand miles."

"Florida!" she says. "Florida!"

G. is in tears again, talking of the angel, whom I see with snow-white wings against a backdrop of Alaskan glacier. "All these people, it's not that they mistreat us"—she is sharp enough to give the staff its due. "But I can't do everything they want, gadding about all over the place. I can't. I wish that angel would come and wrap its wings around me, and just hold me until all this is over."

I share genes with Aunt J.J., not with stepmother G. Mentally I ticket myself for Switzerland, the World Future Conference, thirty years from now. Still, it was G. who, coherent a very few years ago, said to me, "Oh, your fifties are wonderful, wonderful! I never felt better in my life than I did in my fifties. After that it kinda goes downhill."

Do I believe her? I fear I do. I fear. I do. *Over the hill*, what a curiously apt expression after all! The driving and striving slowed, the view superb, you hand off the Sisyphus rock to the person on your left and, if you're lucky enough to have the health, the means, and the inclination, you stroll down the other side of the alp, working with gravity, gravity working with you. But don't relax; your job now is to put on the brakes a little. Power walk. Don't sit in the wheelchair, the wheels will do what wheels are meant to do. The angel is not always there when you need her, and stepdaughters are notoriously off in Florida.

TALE

Everyone has this story, the tale of the Goblin Obgyn, so it will not be necessary to tell it again, right?

No. True stories are only believed with frequent telling. So here is mine, not so long ago and far away:

When I was forty-five my second marriage ended with the end of his fidelity. I had been happy in the marriage, he hadn't gone out looking for an affair, but it had happened, and my trust had not survived. I had already been through divorce once, and this time I handled it, on the whole, pretty well—understanding that it's harder work to leave than to be left, and that it's easier to end a good relationship than a bad one. All the same, after a month or so I began to bleed and didn't stop for three weeks.

I went to my GP, a gentle and personable intern in family practice. I wasn't willing to go back to Dr. B., the obgyn I used to see, I explained, because he had wanted to perform a hysterectomy for no better reason than that, in his opinion, I already had children enough. When I'd told Dr. B. I was not willing to fool around with my psyche in that way, he'd assured me that the loss of a uterus wouldn't bother me. (*Esprit d'escalier:* Shall we cut your balls off then?)

Now Dr. G.P. asked what I was doing to get myself through the divorce. I was keeping busy in the evening, I said, by getting cast in a play. I was recarpeting, for renewal in the house. I was lunching with women friends and driving to the coast every other weekend to be with my younger son in his summer stock company. If I felt I was in trouble, I said, I'd go for counseling.

"People pay thousands of dollars," he cheered me by assuring me, "to learn how to cope like that." All the same, for medical caution, he'd like me to see a gynecologist. There was a new one in town, young, he probably wouldn't give me any nonsense.

At the new Dr. M.'s, the nurse administered a hemoglobin test and stashed me in the cubicle. Dr. M. came in all brisk-and-clipboard and began to take a medical history. I told him ("me and my big mouth" is the self-deprecatory phrase that comes to mind; in fact I think after all these years I am remarkably trusting, and that this is a virtue, not a lack)—why I had not gone back to Dr. B.

"B.'s a good man," he said. "If he wanted to take your womb out, I probably will too." I blanched and held my tongue. When Dr. M. got to the advent, in my medical history, of a second dilation and curettage, he said, "Good lord, two D & Cs. I'm certainly going to take your womb out. I'm not going to start manipulating you with hormones now!"

"No," I agreed, dry. "But I don't think there's anything wrong with my womb. I think I'm under stress. I'm going through a divorce."

"I know, you're depressed and anxious."

"No," I said, "I'm not. I may be later, but at the moment I'm very active, a bit hyper. It's my usual coping pattern."

"You're depressed and anxious," he repeated, as the nurse came in with the test results. "That's funny. Your blood is normal."

"I'm sure it is," I said. "I think this is a normal reaction to stress, and it'll abate of its own accord."

"I'm the doctor," he actually said. "I'm not interested in the total picture, just my specialty, and then we'll slot it *into* the total picture. It's very clear that what you've got here is dysfunctional bleeding, and you'll need a hysterectomy."

Dysfunctional bleeding? Is that a diagnosis? I thought that's the symptom I came in with. Hysterectomy? We cut out my uterus to slot it into the total picture? Is that some form of medical collage? Dr. M., having diagnosed and prescribed, now left me to undress for the pelvic.

I sat for a minute seething. I powerfully did not want to be touched by his immaculate hands. I had a stabbing awareness of the times in my life when I would not have been able to get mad. I thought: Just now it's important for me to feel good about myself. I can't afford the luxury of decorum.

I excused myself to the nurse. "He's made me angry, and I'm not going to have the examination. I'll tell him so myself."

I did so, with surface calm and underrage. The doctor sat rigid in his dignity. I was minutely mollified that he didn't charge me for the blood test.

Two days later I had a call from my ally Dr. G.P. "I got to thinking about you," he said in his pleasant way, "and I thought maybe we ought to set up an appointment with a psychiatrist just to be sure, because, after all, you must be pretty depressed and anxious."

Bewildered, I let him make the appointment, and it was a half hour later that I tumbled to it, how the boys' network works. This had been one of the few times in my life that I acted, clean and immediate, on anger. I wondered, then, about those two D & Cs—were they unnecessary too?—

and about the thousands of wombs that were waved away, this way, from women caught more vulnerable than indignant. I wonder now, having learned that flooding is a sign of the climacteric, which stress my body was undergoing, and when the medical establishment will turn its attention to such matters.

Luckily, the following Tuesday (my bleeding having stopped by then), I was able to convince the psychiatrist that I was sane in spite of my unseemly attachment to my uterus.

STAIR

Beginning in my teens I used to dream of a house through whose stories I descended carrying a baby in my arms. The staircases would lead to doors that opened into rooms that opened into staircases *ad infinitum*. The baby was damaged in some way, clubfooted, or more often, wearing the medieval-painting face of an old man. I loved this offspring dearly, and would wake sad at its imperfection.

In my late forties, I dreamed that I had left the baby in the house in Sussex. I went to retrieve it—her?—but the house was full of strangers, tourists somehow, browsing through bric-a-brac for sale on a flagstone terrace above the lawn. The baby was upstairs, but though I could see the stairs I couldn't get to them. Someone said the baby wouldn't know me, and I was abashed, having no evidence it was otherwise.

One reading offered of dreams in general is that both babies and houses are the self, and I can make sense of that. Young, I felt that I carried my deformed self through the labyrinth of my self; middle-aged, I went to the self I had left behind to find a portion of my self that no longer claimed me.

Another reading offered is that the dream of babies is a dream of ovum, those that can come to fruit and those that remain a thwarted promise in the body. I can make sense of that too, the fearful weight of motherhood and then the poignancy of its loss.

But now I am thinking of the stairs. Between the fear of damaged babies and the regret of no more babies lie thirty-five years of friendship with the woman with whom I have discussed such notions. J. is not my only confidante, but she is the one with whom this particular form of friendship most applies; that we talk the ideas of emotion. We cerebrate about feelings. We are moved by concepts. We analyze impulse. We noeticize sentiment. We fabulate explanation.

And the point is, I never dreamed of friendship. Whatever animal-deep blood-dark feelings rule my dreams, friendship happened gradually in ordinary light. When J. and I met it was a tedious faculty wives' tea. We got together because of trivial judgment on the local restaurants. We spent the first year over Scrabble, embroidery, TV; and have lived in the same town for only one six-month patch since then. Often we were apart for years without a phone call or a note, then took the conversation up midsentence. We ran into each other in London and then it seemed worth the trouble to meet in Belgium, Sussex, Illinois. When I divorced I went where she was. When I went mad she talked me through. When I was happy I discovered that I was telling her the story of my joy. When she went with her family to India I joined them, and we traveled together through Uttar Pradesh ("Oh," she and I still say in praise of each other's clothes, "it's utter pra-desh!"). When we traveled through the climacteric it occurred to us that we'd better not let a year go by without meeting somewhere, and now we do—sometimes alone, sometimes with our men in tow, in rental cars and rural restaurants, all four of us willing to honor the longevity of our friendship.

It's my luck that J. is a family therapist, with a certain amount of codified knowledge about the stuff I write. I offer her fiction's insights too. Years ago she showed me her "stair graph" of intimate relationship. People approach each other in the form of two facing staircases. At first they're far apart on the topmost tread; each takes a tentative step forward, toward the other. Then each descends into herself/himself, and if it seems worth the risk, the effort, takes another step. As long as they keep going into themselves and coming forward, the relationship gets deeper and closer, and can do so till death, though the stairs will never meet. If either refuses either motion, to plumb the self or face the other, the symmetry is skewed and the relationship will strain or break.

We were talking at the time, it will surprise no one to learn, about male-female relationships, and in particular the skewed-asymmetrical-strained quality of my own. The stair graph is a kind of image I can keep in mind even when I am dealing with bifurcating chaos in the gut; and it signally helped me in the area for which she intended it.

Only lately it occurs to me that J. and I, ourselves, have demonstrated her graph, apart and together, delving into our selves and bringing forward what we've found; and that—for all the ova come and gone in our reproductive lives—we've created something that our subconsciouses did not warn us would be the stuff of life. Mating and maternity are in the blood; I have carried babies downstairs and gone upstairs to fetch them both literally and figuratively all the years of my adulthood. But no one is more clearly family to me than J.

In India it happened that we arrived at Fateh pu Sikri on the Feast of Id. I have a snapshot of the two of us, J. and I, backgrounded by the brilliantly silk-swathed stalls, Mutt and Jeff for build, bare-armed and sweating in 110 degrees of Indian July, grinning ourselves toward each other down the ancient steps, old girls in an invented kinship, one step forward, one step down.

HELL

I wake under a feather duvet in a red cover, slightly jetlagged. My stomach is clenched in a sickness of fear, which slowly reveals itself to be attached to something silly, a phone call I have to make, a repair to be seen to. My back aches too, and will never again *not* protest against an overnight airplane seat, so that this connection of travel and pain is a permanent feature remaining to my life. The fear sits sick, and spreads. Something about London, the bombardment from every side of ambition and accomplishment, the failure of socialism, the homeless on the the corner, the posturing of heads of state. My own inadequacy. In a while I will get up, have coffee, do my exercises, have a nice day. Not yet.

In my middle forties I went through a period of two years in which I would wake and rage. The fury was unpredictable in its target. There was always something to attach it to—an imagined slight, a real injustice, an irremediable wound from the past. I resigned myself to the condition as permanent, something I had to endure because it was part of me, probably the fruits of having repressed my anger for so long. Then I stopped drinking alcohol, started taking hormones, and wasn't angry any more.

Now usually I wake with anticipation, admire the plaster rose on my London ceiling or the real banana tree beyond P.'s Florida sliding door, which seems to give off the scent of the coffee he will bring me in a minute. Early-morning moods are rare, and I no longer believe they will outlast the comics page, let alone the calendar. But on the infrequent occasions when the dark ambushes me it is not as anger, but as dread; it takes me by surprise and hits with force.

I have no way of knowing what changes in my body, psyche, spirit, for gain or loss, have to do with menopause, and which have to do with aging, or both, or how much of each. Jet lag, diet, muscle spasm, hormones—I consult the possibilities blind; I recognize recurrent feelings but I can't really judge what comes from situation, what from chemistry. Why should the black mood represent imbalance anyway, instead of simple insight? How much honesty is there in despair? How much of a figment is my usual busy cheer? Here, dark before dawn, muffled in feathers, how much more truth may I touch than in a day of doing?

A statistical analysis on page four of yesterday's *Guardian* shows that pessimistic people have a more realistic view than optimists, both of probabilities and of their own control over events. Optimists, however, *take* better control and therefore accomplish more. Ergo, self-deception is functional.

When I was in my twenties, the fifties, in New York, I bought (from a bargain rack, it must have been, because I was too poor for new hardback books) Katherine Ann Porter's memoir *The Days Before*. The only memory of it I now retain is the pencil-soft portrait on the cover and Porter's observation that we trust hate more than love. Love we think needs to be coaxed and nurtured, carefully maintained. Whereas impulses of contempt have the force of permanent truth. "I love you" is always subject to review. "I hate you" comes from the core.

Mostly, I have taken her observation as admonition. Why should we grant hate such force? Why should we think love so fragile when there's so much evidence of its resilience?

But isn't the answer simply: entropy? Both *eros* and *agape* shatter like a cup knocked on the floor. In some far future when "future" is reversed, the universe contracts, and the past is yet to come, then the cup will jump back on the table and repair itself, hate will need fertilizer pellets, and love will cover the world like kudzu. But I can't imagine such a future, let alone believe in it, and in the meantime affection is fragile, compassion delicate. We are clumsy, ravenous, and short of time.

The image of E. looms as I last saw her, her fierce despair and her cantankerous kindness. We said good-bye on the sill of the Sussex house she was about to lose to taxes, and that was before her paralysis as a writer, before morphine addiction, ten years before she died at ninety-two. My own life may seem to have come round to peace and safety. All the same, the rule is: death.

Abruptly I am off on my death run, worried for my friends, the world. I think X.'s health precarious, and R. lives a gray half-life. Y. may certainly have AIDS. Z. drinks too much, and Q. consumes herself protecting him. How fragile and out of control we are. I would touch wood, but that's too solid. Touch paper, touch leaf, touch cobweb.

I'm surrounded with people (young, but of my own age too) who think the race will muddle through; that sense will solve the population problem, technology restore the rain forests and the ozone layer, goodwill cope with the economy. What evidence supports such hope? Liberal

democracy has triumphed and sells itself like laundry soap. Ethnic auton-
omy turns out to be bloody nationalism. England (England!) is pissing
away its universities. Money represents not production but rumors of
more money. This is not a recision, says J. It is the end of the world as
we've (gluttonously) known it.

Serbia! Sarajevo! We have not given a thought to little Bosnia-
Herzegovina for seventy-eight years, except I understand that the
Orient Express went through, and the rugs were a splendid bargain. Bos-
nian refugees now are being processed through the Austrian camps
through which P. and his family moved after the Second World War. The
lice are still there. "Ethnic cleansing" fights for front-page space with the
incipient collapse of Michael Jackson's plastic face. What do we learn? Are
we worth saving?

Dread floods me like a hot flush. I see this will be one of those days
dogged by clumsiness and tender skin. I will be too large, mincing, mag-
net to objects at the level of my thighs. No, I'll be all right. I'll be better
once I've had coffee, done my exercises, made that call.

Not yet.

HEAL

I have no memory of stepping wrong off a boulder in the Chiricahuas. I
was looking at the canyon, the climb of trees on the other side, the rim
of stones like crumbling columns too tight-packed to fall—and the next
thing I knew I was ass to the ground, one hand around a wrench of pain
in my left ankle and the other clamping a palmful of flesh to the right
knee. I figured the ankle was the more serious but that only an X ray
would see how serious. The knee I took a look at, prizing my hand off
by centimeters.

Pretty bad. The width of my kneecap, a deep scalloped flap like an
upside-down cloud shape, cloud-pale but seeping blood around the
edges—and is that bone, that bit? I'm aware not only of hurt and pound-
ing heart but of incipient and protracted nuisance. Poor P. He'll have to
look after me. He won't mind but I'll be tense with apology. Our poor
vacation, we'll hobble through the rest. Poor me. This is going to take a
long time.

Hand clamped to the knee, blood seeping, I don't realize how long I've
been there until I hear P. calling.

"Jesus, why didn't you yell?"

I'm embarrassed to tell him I was embarrassed to have hurt myself.

It's children who are supposed to be repositories of awe. I don't think so. I think that children accept the natural miracles, and are dazzled only once they have a rudimentary notion of how things work, by things that appear not to—magic, cartoons, fireworks, "effects" that are some way "special." I know that when I was little and skinned my knee, I took it as no great gift that the wound would sting and bleed. I endured the knowledge that my mother would get the dirt out whether I screamed about it or was brave. I knew it would stanch, and scab, and itch, and knit itself, probably with a little scar.

At fifty-five I watch this process with exploding wonder. It happens at wizard speed. The ankle produces its egg swelling within a couple of hours. I can walk on it next day, well enough to perambulate the border into Mexico, to shop for trinkets including a handsome carved cane. It's clear after all no bone is broken, and over the weeks as the swelling recedes it leaves a ring of delicate blue posies around my heel, which gradually like posies fade. The cut is an angry ruck of skin, which sucks itself back to its bed so hard that bending the knee becomes my major problem. I find I am fighting not the hurt but the healing, stretching against the eagerness of my flesh to knit. The blood fists into a dark scab, goes drab, and begins to lift around the edges. The shallower cut at each side of the kneecap smooths and flattens. Within a month, back in Florida in tepid Gulf saltwater, I lose the scab and emerge from the ocean whole, just a slight double-raised pink bloom on my knee, which looks a little tender, though it isn't.

My question is: Why—when, even after a half-century, and after its ability to reproduce itself is past, a body not particularly well looked after will demonstrate its enthusiasm for survival in such wise, will speed good about the veins, pump blood and antibodies, set itself to coagulation, osmosis, cleansing, and creation, will mend so thoroughly that mobility and convenience are restored that could not be had from a half a ton of technology—why, I say, should I ever have bitterly blamed it for such trifles as I have blamed it for: for having too much flesh in this spot, too little muscle in that, for producing this wrinkle, that sag, that gray hair, or this texture? Dear body! My dear body! It has gone about its incessant business with very little thanks.

I wake from a dream of D. We are having tea in a pleasantly shabby Victorian room, books and papers jumbled everywhere. "What are you going to do next?" I asked, and she said, "Nothing."

"Ah," I was a little disconcerted.

"Yes," she said. "I worked so hard early on that I feel I was cheated of my youth. What would you do, if you were going to make up for a lost youth?"

She seemed to want my answer. "I'd get a good masseur," I said. "I'd have a good hard workout, and then a really deep massage."

"I never thought of that." She paid me a look of keen attention.

"Yes, and then I'd dance. I'd read of course, and so forth. But definitely I'd dance."

Waking, I know that I've been blatantly giving me good advice in my sleep. I giggle, reach my fingers out in a balletic gesture, meaning to touch P.'s back, but my forearm tumbles off the edge of the single bed, into the void under the red duvet. Oh yes. Another week before I'm back in Florida.

Okay. A week of friends and work. My ceiling rose is very pretty. I wrap myself for comfort, and in the hazy sleeplight I remember another quilt, the blue chintz with the cotton satin border that my grandmother made when I was—six? It was kapok-filled, the stuffing held in place by yarn ties; I remember her plumb fingers pulling tight the knots.

There is a photograph of me on the quilt, spread on the spiky brown grass in front of the house on Alvarado Street. I am on my stomach, arms stiff in front of me, pointed toe touching my forehead over my arched back. I am ringletted like Shirley Temple, wearing a blue ruffled satin dance dress with tiny straps.

I remember too the buying of that costume, a miracle out of a rummage sale, one sleepy dawn when there was still such a thing as a vacant lot in downtown Phoenix, and the Women's Society for Christian Service had filled it with church tables covered in white paper and old clothes. I wandered among the rows while my mother sorted castoffs that Black and Mexican women waited in the hot dark to buy, for small change that the church would send to Africa.

I remember discovering the satin slip of a ruffled dress, pulling it out of a jumble of plaid cotton and scratchy wools. I remember my fear that some other mother would buy it before I could convince my own; and the hot quarter mom slipped into my palm, which I handed over to the church lady behind the table; for satin, for ruffles. For a snapshot of a pose on the chintz quilt.

There are also photographs of me in pastel taffeta for the Gene Bumph revue, with silver sparkles on the yoke and a tilted pancake hat held in place by tight elastic; in a variegated fall of silk chiffon-turquoise, azure, emerald—when I danced a piece of seaweed to Ruth St. Denis's octopus; in patent leather tap shoes with glossy bows and silver heels;

in a pink tutu; in a red satin bum-skimmer skirt with white band jacket, gold lurex frogs.

How I wanted to dance! And how persistently my body announced itself unfit for such endeavor. Apologizing for the extravagance of my lessons, Mom would laugh, "I've got to do something about her, she's so clumsy!" Nor did this register as a cruelty, for I also thought our mutual desire was hubris. I was the stage child of a stage mother. I sat in the dark recital halls and made Shirley Temple moues.

At home my brother grunted while I practiced acrobatics on the living room rug. Chest rolls, backbends. Amos 'n' Andy played on the radio; Dad sat at once inert and intent, because he loved a good "show." My mother darned. I did headstands with my head on a cushion and my hands positioned for a tripod; I did elbow stands with my soles against the door, while my brother sat on the couch mocking, saying: *Ugh! I can do that too!*

There were toe shoes, little wads of lambswool, pain; and the satin ribbons crossed up my calves frenetically, as if I could will myself into a *prima.* There was a sheer rig in an autumnal theme, in the synthetics that had come in by then, skimpy on my solid prepubescent frame. There was the hateful, garish jester's costume when I became too thick for acrobatics and was cast as the physical equivalent of a straight man in what they dignified with the name "Adagio."

Wrong body, wrong body. I gave up the lessons, finally. I went to the North High basketball dance and stood in a corner in flocked nylon, praying for anybody to ask me onto the floor. I learned to jitterbug, defiant, and took a prize at it with my brother's college roommate. I learned to twist in time to chaperon my first college students. Once, in my thirties, I hired a teacher for a party, for a lark, during the disco phase.

My body, my poor body. When was it I learned to put on a tape and dance for me?

I stretch my ankle into a gingerly *point,* finger the polished scar. I think: Dying, we heal. Over the hill, both body and psyche are still scrambling after order for themselves.

I know this. I learned very late why my love affairs ended in diminishment and recrimination. It's a long story that I can tell in a phrase or two. I always chose men I could not please. I worked very hard to understand this, and finally I understood it. I worked very hard to change, and eventually I changed. Bit by bit my psyche coagulated, scabbed and knit.

Now I bend my knee, caress its fresh bloom. The costumes turn in my mind, cutouts of photographs, afloat. They tumble around me in a slow

free fall. They are all there, the bows and the spangles, the chiffons waiting, the satin ruffles; they are putting me back to sleep. My duvet lifts and
begins to lose its color. It pales and floats as a cloud would float, unsup-
ported in the middle air. Around me, Chagall-like, Aunt J.J. and W. go
power walking on a nimbus. G.'s wheelchair spins. J. is skipping down a
stair, E. is rocking back and forth over her Sussex sill. The world's a long
way down.

I learned an interesting fact about detachment. Apparently the reason
leaves fall is that as summer ends they suddenly produce a burst of fresh
growth. They're so productive that the join at the matrix near the branch
is weak. Then even a slight wind will break them off.

J. said that older people find it necessary to detach, and do so in myr-
iad ways. They get deaf, they don't remember. They relive their lives, go
quiet, go inward, concentrating on self. Dying and healing in tandem,
they go about the natural, necessary business of letting go.

This process is hardly begun in me. I have loving yet to do. But I know
what it means, I feel the beginning of it, on my cloud duvet. I have nearly
learned that I can't control what happens in the world. I've nearly understood that I don't have to. I have nearly got it, that my friends and I are
going to die, and that whether the planet offs itself will be decided without particular reference to me. I can do a little, and I'm responsible for
the little I can do. I can give X. a call tomorrow, recycle my trash, for
instance. I can value P. and celebrate my scar.

That's all. That's all I can do, and all I am required to do. In the gray
half-light of sleep I climb my duvet to dance.

FAYE MOSKOWITZ

The Matriarchs Grow Old, My Models

◈

The matriarchs grow old, my models, women who were women when I was a child. Who will be left to call me "Faygele" when they are no longer here? With no one but me to recall my childhood, who will validate the memories? They will carry pieces of me when they go. How much of their strength will they bequeath to me? The years pass, and the distance between us collapses in fan folds; one day I will be standing where they are now. . . .

Home, after work, I turn on the answering machine, pen in hand, to note the names and numbers. A buzz, and then Aunt Lena's voice floats out of the recorder, no ear to cup the sound before it fills the room. "I'm sorry to be the one to tell you this," she begins, and I feel defenseless, somehow, against the disembodied message. "Aunt Rachel passed away last night," she says. Where are the muffled drumbeats, the clamor of bells? Only this scratchy old-time radio voice, trapped in vinyl tape.

I call my husband to impart the news, discuss with him the best way to inform his aged mother that her sister-in-law is dead. His mother has had a hard winter, and we are fearful of jarring her fragile equilibrium. We decide to tell her at dinner, the first time we will be together again that day.

Seated at the table, we avoid her eyes, drop our glances away from the shaking hands, attenuate the time until the announcement. It hurts to imagine how she must feel, on the firing line of old age, wondering if she will be the next to fall. "Let's get it over with," my husband mutters. His mother doesn't hear him; she is quite deaf.

I will be the one to say it, I tell myself. Perhaps I can phrase the words more gently than he can. But I quail at the deafness, the problem of delivering bad news at the top of my lungs. The possibility of nuance is gone;

I cannot soften the harsh words by a lowering of the voice or the gloss of inflection.

"Ma," I say, at last, raising my voice, "Rachel passed away; Aunt Lena called." The piece of bread is halfway to her mouth, and she continues to carry it in one unbroken sweep. "Tough woman," my husband says of his aunt. "Rachel was a cossack!" his mother affirms. I look her full in the face now. She is dry-eyed, a tough woman, too.

I wonder how tough *I* am, now that the years stretch behind me in a swath sufficient to reveal texture and design. Are there surprises left? My responses seem to me these days as predictable as the tobacco-covered pennies that turn up at the bottom of my purse. The women of whom I speak: their lives were tempered by pogroms, the blast from gas ovens. They endured loss of land and language, answered to "green horn" before they knew what the term meant. By contrast with them, my life has reached the softball stage in the likes of a jelly kettle. I pray I never endure their crucible, but I covet the nature of their strength. . . .

The world tastes flat—meat without salt, more often than not. I know how fortunate I am to have been born in my own special time and place. Still, that doesn't cheer me when I get the blues any more than the example of starving babies in China ever made leftover food more palatable when I was a child. I ponder the years to come and see mixed messages everywhere I go. . . .

Three elderly ladies share a bench at the neighborhood supermarket, crocheted shopping bags and metal carts tucked at their sides. Dressed for the season, they sport dark, flowered polyester dresses, good wool coats, and tidy hats. The few minutes of gossip they exchange add importance to an errand already blown out of proportion by the meagerness of their days.

A similarly clad shopper passes the seated group and calls to one of the bench warmers. "Hi, neighbor," she says. A blank look for response, and then, "Why! I didn't recognize you!" Halfway to the exit, the first calls back crisply, "You never do." "Well," says the seated neighbor in self-defense, "You've changed so." Shoulders slumping, the departing woman mumbles to no one in particular, "Don't I know it!"

At fifty-two, I feel changes also. Not since my teens, the years when we are all eager for the clock to speed up, have birthdays provoked such introspection. I was conscious of the passage of time back then in a way the intervening years have never mirrored. Too busy, perhaps, bearing babies, raising them, finally growing up myself, to watch the clock.

For a long time, I approached birthdays calmly, counting out the com-

fortable number of years I could reasonably expect according to the bib-
lical formula (as good a measure as any), and always the three score and
ten allowed me more than half of what I had already eaten up. After I
reached the "halfway" mark, I changed the rules and began to measure by
actuarial tables; still there was comfort in the numbers. Now, add and
subtract as I may, the balance is against me. I find more years gone by than
I can hope to have in store.

For the first time, I wish I had some of those years to live over again.
That beautiful decade between forty and fifty: I wouldn't waste it sleeping so much, dreaming, staring at walls, doing crossword puzzles, listening to the stories of people I don't really care very much about. Things are
different now that the moon is no longer my timekeeper. The depressions
can't be so easily explained away by a knowing glance at the calendar. I
wonder if I have time left to write a novel; will I ever shape the hoarded
bits of brightly colored fabric into the quilt I have always thought I'd
make one day?

The hair I swore I'd never cut, "until I die," I playfully said, hangs
heavy, makes me question long-range promises. My daughter told me
tactfully not long ago, "They have great hair coloring now; you should
really think about it." I do. My students beg me to let my hair hang loose
instead of bound in a knot, and I brush them away like insistent flies. I
don't want to look like the women I see in the country with Dolly Par-
ton pompadours and sagging faces underneath. Nevertheless, I understand about outer changes. What the poet Robert Frost calls "inner
weather" concerns me more.

The days whirl by in a rhythm of their own, freewheeling, out of my
control. I grab at the nights with my fingertips and cannot hold on. Be
productive, I tell myself, not certain any longer just what my quota is. I
write, I teach, I mother and wife, I eat and drink and read. But my shadow
shortens and threatens to catch up with me. I look to the matriarchs for
their secrets and see they are falling. They speak to me with words that
echo Eliot's *Wasteland.* "HURRY UP," they say. "HURRY UP PLEASE, IT'S
TIME."

BONNIE BRAENDLIN

Mrs. Ramsay, Menopause and Me:
A Reading of Virginia Woolf's
To the Lighthouse

✠

Asked to give the banquet speech at the (primarily male) Western Gerontological Association Convention in Albuquerque, New Mexico, in 1983, I queried mildly, "Why can't men age more like women?" A few of the women took me aside afterward to tell me, with great amusement, how I had threatened the men. They themselves had loved it.

"But why were the men uncomfortable?" I asked. "I didn't attack them. I deliberately stayed away from feminist issues."

"It wasn't your feminism," one of the women said. "You were so *personal*. You talked about their *own* aging. That's not the way it's done in gerontology."

Betty Friedan, *The Fountain of Age*

The menopausal woman is the prisoner of a stereotype and will not be rescued from it until she has begun to tell her own story.

Germaine Greer, *The Change: Women, Aging and the Menopause*

Virginia Woolf's 1927 novel *To the Lighthouse* tells the story of two women—Mrs. Ramsay and Lily Briscoe, the first a wife and mother of eight children, the second an unmarried aspiring artist. The first section depicts the Ramsay family and numerous friends, including Lily, on a summer holiday in the Hebrides before the Great European War. Here Mr. and Mrs. Ramsay argue about a proposed trip to the lighthouse on a nearby island in a running disagreement that epitomizes a marriage between a rational, intellectual, professional male and an emotional, domesticated woman, holdovers from Victorian stereotypes. Ten years pass in the second section, which describes the decay of the Ramsay's

90

summer house in the context of cataclysmic social change precipitated by the war; the third section delineates the return to the Hebrides of Mr. Ramsay, Lily, two of the children and a few friends after Mrs. Ramsay's death, where Lily agonizes over and finally makes her decision to become a professional artist.

Years ago when I first began to teach the novel I identified with and thus centered class discussions on Lily Briscoe and her self-development process as a representation of the early twentieth-century "New Woman" artist. I agreed with critics who interpret Lily as a daughter figure trying to escape the fate of her nineteenth-century surrogate mother, Mrs. Ramsay, the epitome of the wife-mother icon, the Angel in the House. Woolf herself writes in her essay "Professions for Women" that "[k]illing the Angel in the House was part of the occupation of a woman writer. . . . Had I not killed her she would have killed me. She would have plucked the heart out of my writing." I envisioned Mrs. Ramsay, the quintessential matchmaker, as my own mother, telling me that I would be happy if I, nearing thirty and still single, would just marry and have children, when I was eager to advance in academe. Clearly Mrs. Ramsay had to go, and in discussion after discussion with students, I—like Virginia Woolf and without qualms—"took up the inkpot and flung it at her."[1] Over the years I continued to view Lily Briscoe as the protagonist, even as I moved from being primarily a daughter to being a wife and mother, but not identifying with Mrs. Ramsay because in the era of Women's Liberation, I was combining career with marriage. Married at twenty-eight (just in the nick of time, my mother said), I followed my husband from California to his new teaching position in Florida, where I enrolled in graduate school and had a baby; it took me eight years to get the Ph.D., writing my dissertation with one hand and caring for our daughter with the other. As I continued to teach *To the Lighthouse* in a new era of female freedom, I focused even more firmly on Lily as the prototype of a liberated woman. Over the years, as my daughter grew up and went away to college, I played a modern Mrs. Ramsay–Lily Briscoe role: on the one hand, taking my turn at carpooling, cheering my daughter on at swim meets, and presiding at modest but creatively delicious dinners with friends and family, and on the other, teaching university students, supervising teaching assistants, and writing scholarly articles. Never, however, did I feel or convey to my literature students one iota of sympathy or understanding for Mrs. Ramsay as a wife-mother caught in a role not of her own making; continuing to view her as a suffocating surrogate mother for the struggling female artist, I, in effect, continued to pelt her with the inkpot. It was only years later—last year, in fact, when I began to have symptoms finally diagnosed by my gynecologist as menopausal—that I began to understand what Woolf meant when she wrote about the Angel, "She died hard. . . . She was always creeping back when I thought I had despatched her" (PW 1385).

Excerpt from my menopause diary:
My first hot flash begins sometime in the night, somewhere in mid-solar plexus, radiating out along my nerves, lifting me off the bed and floating me in mid-air. Wow, what was that?! The next morning I jump out of bed, alert, hyper, taut as our long, lean cat, George. Before breakfast, before coffee, before the sun is up, I type away at my computer, composing the article that's due in two days, writing more than I've written in weeks. I conduct my classes like a maestro, dash to the library for some research texts I haven't had time to investigate, manage to stay awake during a late-afternoon faculty meeting, cook a decent if not inspired meal, but then suddenly collapse as my husband washes up the dishes. Ten minutes into the nightly rerun of "Murder, She Wrote," I've nodded off; ebbing and flowing in and out of sleep, I try to watch my favorite comedienne and one of the new police shows. Not tonight, all is a blur, and at ten I stagger off to bed, where I sleep soundly for three or four hours before I'm flashed awake again.

One day last year (perhaps it was a day when I was having hot flashes and denying them by playing with the thermostat and asking my students, "Is it *hot* in here or is it just me?"), I suddenly realized, while teaching *To the Lighthouse,* that Mrs. Ramsay had crept back with a vengeance and that she, at fifty, was *I*—or rather, I was identifying with *her*—and we were both *menopausal women,* an epithet, a concept, and a subject position more denigrated and resisted in my culture than the Angel in the House was in Woolf's. At age fifty-three I for some months had been undergoing "the Change"—in Gail Sheehy's words "the Silent Passage"—an unspoken and unsung phase of female self-development, and by throwing the inkpot at Mrs. Ramsay, I was hurling it at myself. In a (hot) flash I shifted my interpretive interest from Lily to Mrs. Ramsay.

As is well known from Woolf's diary entries, Mrs. Ramsay is an imaginary re-creation of Woolf's own mother, who died when she was thirteen; Woolf believed herself to have exorcised her obsession with the dead mother through this portrait. Mrs. Ramsay also epitomizes the Victorian Angel in the House that haunted Woolf's struggle to become a writer. As a version of the "Eternal Feminine" that migrates from Goethe's Germany to nineteenth-century England, where it shows up in

Coventry Patmore's poem *The Angel in the House,* this trope embodies virtues of self-sacrifice, "self-less innocence," and devotion to the needs of a male.[2] The Angel, Woolf writes, is "immensely charming . . . utterly unselfish . . . excell[ing] in the difficult arts of family life . . . [and] sacrific[ing] herself daily" (PN 1385). These traits describe Mrs. Ramsay to a "T": she is the consummate self-sacrificing woman, fleshing out the mystique of wife-motherhood, an embodiment of beauty, love, warmth, fecundity, domestic creativity, maternal comfort and charity. Most men, except for the eccentric poet Mr. Carmichael, fall in love with her beauty and elevate her to goddess status. The young atheist Tansley realizes in an epiphanic moment that "she was the most beautiful person he had ever seen." Indeed, her beauty inspires him to an uncharacteristic outburst: "With stars in her eyes and veils in her hair, with cyclamen and wild violets—what nonsense was he thinking."[3] Even after many years of marriage, Mr. Ramsay, "bending his magnificent head before her . . . does homage to the beauty of the world" (TTL 36). When her husband, insecure in his own aging process, demands sympathy, she becomes for him a sensual and energizing "rain of energy," a "delicious fecundity," a "fountain and spray of life" (TTL 37). Although she appears to favor her youngest son, James, Mrs. Ramsay exhibits maternal concern for all her eight children, appreciating and nurturing each one's individual talents and abilities. At age fifty, as a devoted wife of a devoted husband and a solicitous mother of adoring children, Mrs. Ramsay appears to be a version of ideal middle-aged womanhood, beautiful, beloved, beatific, blessed.

Yet Mrs. Ramsay is not entirely a happy, fulfilled Angel; sometimes she is at least vaguely discontented with this role and questions its "selflessness": "For her own self-satisfaction was it that she wished so instinctively to help, to give, that people might say of her, 'O Mrs. Ramsay! dear Mrs. Ramsay . . . Mrs. Ramsay, of course!' and need her and send for her and admire her?" (TTL 42). On the one hand, she recognizes "the torch of her beauty" and that because of it and her unselfish devotion to the needs of others, "[s]he had been admired. She had been loved"; but at the same time, she realizes she is: "[s]habby and worn out, and not presumably (her cheeks were hollow, her hair was white) any longer a sight that filled the eyes with joy" (TTL 41–2). Here Mrs. Ramsay teeters on the brink of menopausal awareness, a condition described thus by Germaine Greer: "Sooner or later the middle-aged woman becomes aware of a change in the attitude of other people towards her. She can no longer trade on her appearance, something which she has done unconsciously all her life" (TC 8). Mrs. Ramsay is occasionally bewildered by her self-sacrificing life: "Not that she herself was 'pessimistic,' as [her husband] accused her of being. Only she thought life—and a little strip of time presented itself to her eyes—her fifty years. There it was before her—life. Life, she thought—but she did not finish her thought" (TTL 59). At one point Mrs. Ramsay even acknowledges that life, like her busy day, "had slipped past in one quick doing after another" and was "ephemeral as a rainbow"(TTL16).

Excerpt from my menopause diary:
The most amazing symptom of menopause is that I'm able to stop time; not literally of course, well, literally in a way because every time I take my Swiss Army Watch off my wrist it ticks away for a few minutes, then the second hand jerks back and forth a few times before stopping dead in its tracks. Last summer in Switzerland I took it to a watch repair shop but they were baffled. No, *nein, non madame,* it doesn't need a new battery, they shook their heads in agreement but could come up with no cure, not even a reasonable assessment of the possible problem. Only later did I begin to realize that the watch was charged with my new energy. Now my "menopause trick" is a hit at parties, dinners, any place where people (perhaps after a few drinks) are happy to be entertained when the conversation lags. "My watch stops shortly after I remove it from my wrist," I tell them, "and it won't run again until I put it back on." The more sophisticated among them raise eyebrows or feign disinterest, but inevitably everyone's interest is piqued when, sure enough, five or six minutes after I take it off, the watch stops. Some pick it up and try it on, and for some it works (particularly for those women and men close to my age, I note with glee), but most just shrug or smile and hand it back to me. "It's my menopausal zest," I grin, "my new power as the crone; I now control chronological time, and . . . since I've kept you entertained for some time, psychological time as well!"

While Mrs. Ramsay, unlike Greer's hypothetical menopausal woman, *does* "continue living [her] life mainly through responses to the needs of those in [her] household" (TC 40), she occasionally resents her compliance: "She often felt she was nothing but a sponge sopped full of human emotions" (TTL 32). She also resists self-effacement by "no longer suppress[ing her] own curiosities, and [her] own insights and opinions, in order to let other people express theirs" (TC 40), or at least not entirely. But when she tries to express an opinion, others, especially her children, laugh at her, thus locking her more securely into the Angel role. In moments alone, however, after the children are in bed, Mrs. Ramsay indulges in a desire for individuality that she suppresses during her daily devotion to other's needs: "She could be herself, by herself. And that was what now she often felt the need of. . . . To be silent; to be alone . . . a wedge-shaped core of darkness, something invisible to others" (TTL 62). Here she appears to be in the first stage of a rite of passage, defined by Ann Mankowitz as one "of isolation, withdrawal of the individual from society and into close contact with, and dependence upon, nature."[4] That it is a menopausal rite of passage is suggested by the fact that Mrs. Ramsay is fifty and apparently past child-bearing age, her youngest children, James and Cam, being six and seven years old. She may be seen as exemplifying Greer's description of the menopausal woman in search of something other than Angelhood: "Poets since classical times have celebrated an ideal stage of tranquil thoughtfulness to round off a busy life. The woman of fifty has even more reason to long for that time; after menopause, when she may be permitted to give up being someone's daughter, someone's love, someone's wife and someone's mother, she may also be allowed to turn into herself" (TC 40).

Mood swings, that staple of menopausal ideology, are a part of Mrs. Ramsay's life. At the epitome of her performance as wife-mother at the dinner party, when Prue locks her into an other-defined identity—"That's my mother"—"[i]nstantly, for no reason at all, Mrs. Ramsay became like a girl of twenty, full of gaiety. A mood of revelry suddenly took possession of her." Here she teeters on the brink of selfish desire, wishing to join the young people in a spontaneous walk to the beach to "watch the waves" (TTL 116), a frivolous and self-satisfying act that would be a defiant act for a traditional woman. But the desire for a youthful escape is soon brought back into control by an internalized compulsion to duty, and Mrs. Ramsay finds herself "withheld by something so strong that she never even thought of asking herself what it was. Of course it was impossible for her to go with them . . . and tickled by the absurdity of her thought . . . she went with a smile on her lips into the other room, where her husband sat reading" (TTL 117).

Mrs. Ramsay does not pursue modes of action and reaction that Greer sees as marking the resistant menopausal woman: She does not, for example, please herself by choosing which jewelry to wear down to dinner, as she might do according to Greer's conjecture about "the new attitude of older women to jewelry"; instead she lets her children choose for her. Neither does she "declare a taste for her own tipple . . . on the drinks tray" (TC 50), but then eating, not drinking, is the mode of consumption in Woolf's novel. At her famous dinner party Mrs. Ramsay seems to be the perfect hostess, helping her guests to the best pieces of meat and making sure that Mr. Carmichael gets a second helping of soup. But this gesture of hospitality also defies Mr. Ramsay's annoyance at Carmichael's request and thus may be a sign of resistance in the House Angel. The dinner party scene, where Mrs. Ramsay tries to harmonize the discordant voices in her household, is the high point of her domestic creativity. As she lights the candles that unite her diners, she unifies them in a brief moment of timelessness, watched over by herself as "a hawk suspended; like a flag [she] floated in an element of joy which filled every nerve of her body fully and sweetly, not noisily, solemnly rather, for it arose, she thought, looking at them all eating there, from husband and children and friends . . . holding them safe together. . . . It partook, she felt . . . of eternity. . . . Of such moments, she thought, the thing is made that endures" (TTL 105).

Excerpt from my menopause diary:
At a buffet dinner in the home of a colleague, my husband and I mingle with others of our ilk, university professors and their spouses, chatting about our kids and the latest academic gossip. Two young women sit all evening on the sofa, their slim bodies almost entwined, the fashionable, discreet décolletages and decorously long skirts revealing everything and nothing. The older women, myself included, glance at them fondly and rather patronizingly, although they are, in addition to being faculty wives, also assistant professors, schooled at the best universities and already well published. Most of the men congregate by the buffet, swapping stories of travels in Europe, computer buys, and the perils of owning ancient Volvos and Volkswagens; they glance covertly at the young professor-wives whenever they lean forward to fetch their wine glasses from the coffee table or cross and uncross their shapely legs in a swirl of chiffon. Alert young non-academic wives glare at the men; we older wives cast furtive glances toward our husbands, but, having played this scene many times, we immediately revert back to our own conversations. The beautiful young professor-wives remain oblivious to the male gazes, deep in earnest discussions apparently of no importance to anyone but themselves.

Our hostess, an Asian Mrs. Ramsay in an elegant gold and red tunic, weaves back and forth between the dining room buffet, resplendent with Chinese delicacies, and her dinner guests, urging us to fill our plates over and over in a ritual of gluttonous overindulgence.

"I went menopausal this year," I say to a longtime acquaintance, the wife of a department chairman, herself a sculptor of some local renown. "Oh my," she replies, almost involuntarily, raising her eyebrows slightly. I sense that she is uneasy with this topic, but intrigued as well. "Are you on hormones?" she ventures cautiously, then seeing me shake my head, she blurts out, "Good!"

"I waited a year before going to my gynecologist because I knew he would insist on hormones," I tell her. "As it was, I had to keep insisting that I wanted to try without them. I exercise, lift weights, take calcium—all the things that supposedly help alleviate menopausal symptoms, so I don't want to take anything. Finally he said, 'Well, I guess it would be a waste of my time to write you a prescription. You probably wouldn't have it filled anyway.'"

We both laugh at this, although I can feel at the back of my head or in my gut a tiny nagging doubt. What if the doctors are right? What about osteoporosis? Heart disease?

While Mrs. Ramsay has often been characterized as an artist of human relations, exemplified by her facility at keeping the conversation going at dinner, her actions and perceptions regarding the fruit bowl suggest that she is an incipient aesthetic artist as well: "Indeed she had been keeping guard over the dish of fruit (without realizing it) jealously, hoping that nobody would touch it. Her eyes had been going in and out among the curves and shadows of the fruit, among the rich purples of the lowland grapes, then over the horny ridge of the shell, putting a yellow against a purple, a curved shape against a round shape, without knowing why she did it, or why, every time she did it, she felt more and more serene" (TTL 108–9). Her insistence on keeping the fruit centerpiece intact as a work of art suggests that she subconsciously desires to be an artist, a profession that in her day was mutually exclusive with being a wife-mother. Ironically, perhaps, the Angel who tempted Lily (and by extension, Woolf herself) to that role and away from art, may herself have wished to be an artist.

Only to herself does Mrs. Ramsay admit to the desire for another calling, a move into the New Woman position: "She ruminated the other problem, of rich and poor, and the things she saw with her own eyes, weekly, daily, here or in London, when she visited this widow, or that struggling wife in person with a bag on her arm, and a note-book and pencil with which she wrote down in columns carefully ruled for the purpose wages and spending, employment and unemployment, in the hope that thus she would cease to be a private woman whose charity was half a sop to her own indignation, half a relief to her own curiosity, and become what with her untrained mind she greatly admired, an investigator, elucidating the social problem" (TTL 9). Mrs. Ramsay, however, does not renounce home and family, nor does she fulfill her vague dreams of becoming an artist or a social worker. Firmly ensconced as the Angel in her house, Mrs. Ramsay rebels only in a passive-aggressive way when she refuses to declare her love for her husband, while knowing that he knows she loves him.

Most readers at the time *To the Lighthouse* appeared, if they recognized Mrs. Ramsay as menopausal, probably would have considered her condition to be debilitating: "From the turn of the century, when the word 'menopause' began to figure in medical literature, the notion that the climacteric was a time of mental and physical derangement became one of the things that everybody knew" (TC 24). Woolf was not menopausal at the time she wrote the novel, but indications from her diary ten years later are that she also regarded menopause as an illness, one that she likens to her own bouts of insanity, identified by scholars today as bi-polar disorder. On Monday, March 1, 1937, when Woolf was fifty-five years old, she wrote, "I wish I could write out my sensations at this moment. They are so peculiar and so unpleasant. Partly T. of L. [time of life, a euphemism, for menopause]." And on March 2 she pleaded, "Suffer me now and again to write out my horror, this sudden cold madness, here. It is partly T. of L. I think still."[5] But whether Mrs. Ramsay would become deranged or rebellious in her menopause is a moot question, for in the second section of the novel, Woolf kills the Angel that haunted her, "Mr. Ramsay, stumbling along a passage one dark morning, stretched his arms out, but Mrs. Ramsay having died rather suddenly the night before, his arms, though stretched out, remained empty" (TTL 128).

In my menopausal mind, however, Mrs. Ramsay remains a resistant icon.

Excerpt from a letter written by my friend Judy:
At forty-five, menopausal, and suffering from hormonal & chemical imbalances in my own life, I feel as if I am in a novel, a nightmarish one, where life is changing faster than I can keep up with it. The tables have turned & I have found myself offering guidance to my parents. Also, at other times they become the child & I the adult as they throw tantrums. *Mid Life.* In my own case I have a wonderful gyn. who has me on hormones to help with mood swings, hot flashes, and most of all migraines that set in as soon as perimenopause did. The migraines are being managed as is depression. Turning forty turned my life inside out. I am now seeing the benefits of hormonally & chemically balancing my body.

Thank God it is 1994 and assertive women have cared *not* to suffer as our mothers did in what my mother still will only call "the change."

Reading Judy's letter it occurs to me that Lily Briscoe, age forty-four in the last section of *To the Lighthouse*, is not too young to be menopausal. In addition to representing the New Woman of her day, who chooses the artistic life over the domestic, she may also be read as a reincarnation of her surrogate mother, Mrs. Ramsay, whose energy and creativity she recovers in memory and absorbs as her own: "'Mrs. Ramsay!' Lily cried, 'Mrs. Ramsay!' . . . It was strange how clearly she saw her, stepping with her usual quickness across fields among whose folds, purplish and soft, among whose flowers, hyacinths or lilies, she vanished. It was some trick of the painter's eye. For days after she had heard of her death she had seen her thus, putting her wreath to her forehead and going unquestioningly with her companion, a shade across the fields. The sight, the phrase, had its power to console. Wherever she happened to be, painting, here, in the country or in London, the vision would come to her, and her eyes, half closing, sought something to base her vision on" (TTL 181). By incorporating Mrs. Ramsay into her art and in so doing finding her artistic vision, Lily Briscoe may fulfill the menopausal rite of passage as a quest for self-defined identity.

But that's another story for another time and place.

ENDNOTES

1. "Professions for Women," *The Norton Anthology of Literature by Women.* Ed. Sandra M. Gilbert and Susan Gubar (NY: Norton 1985) 1385. Hereafter cited in the text as PW.
2. Sandra M. Gilbert and Susan Gubar. *The Madwoman in the Attic: The Woman Writer and the Nineteenth-Century Literary Imagination* (New Haven and London: Yale UP 1979) 21–23.
3. Virginia Woolf. *To the Lighthouse.* Foreword by Eudora Welty. (San Diego, NY, London: Harcourt Brace Jovanovich 1989.) Hereafter cited in the text as TTL.
4. Quoted by Germaine Greer. *The Change: Women, Aging and the Menopause* (NY: Fawcett Columbine 1991) 36. Hereafter cited in the text as TC.
5. Quoted in Quentin Bell, *Virginia Woolf: A Biography* (NY: Harcourt Brace Jovanovich 1972) 198–99.

SUSAN TERRIS

Flesh

✠

When I pinch it, a ridge of faded peach faille
slowly flattens out.
Once, it resembled skin of the sleeping newborn
crooked in my elbow: satiny,
sensuous to the touch.
Today, scarred, pocked and stencilled, it forms
porous, rippled plains. Just when I came to enjoy
it, modeled like a sleek self-shawl, it began
to stretch, creping topographical maps
along neck and arms.
Now veins river them, river my legs, too.
Shirred rosettes dot my hands; and when I fist
them, knobs of bone project.
That bone with its pallor suggests mortality,
the whited bone and sack of skin which,
long before death, was my husband's mother.
Lift her and she caved in as though,
over time, she'd forgotten her imprint.

But I recall mine; so when the baby, my grandson,
awakens, I—stirred by archaic impulses—
unbutton, unhook and respond.
Cupping my teat, I edge it toward his mouth.
As he latches on, the half-remembered
pull and clamp unnerve me.
Oblivious to my agitation, the child burrows

into damp flesh.
Then abruptly, he arches, rears his head,
outraged, aware he has been tendered a sham:
no firmness, no lushness, no milk.
I, similarly outraged, match him howl for howl.

MARY ELSIE ROBERTSON

Change of Life

❈

When I was growing up in Arkansas in the forties and fifties, the "change of life" was spoken of in hushed tones and never mentioned in mixed company. The women who came to visit my mother on hot summer mornings helped her peel peaches or shell peas while they spoke—in the same near whisper they would have used talking about some unmarried girl in the town getting pregnant—of Hettie Jenks or Cass O'Bar or Cora Ford, who had reached her change of life and was finding it hard to bear.

I played quietly in my corner with my paper dolls, careful not to draw attention to myself since I knew my mother would send me outside to play if she remembered I was in the room. So I certainly couldn't ask a question from my corner, though I had no idea what the "change of life" was. The only change of life I knew about occurred in fairy stories in which a brother might be turned into a deer or a frog suddenly become a handsome prince. Many of the changes that occurred to the people in stories were desirable ones—the handsome prince would, I assumed, rather be a prince than a frog—but I knew by the tone of the women's voices in my mother's kitchen that the change of life they were talking about was an undesirable and even frightening one. A woman could, I gathered, lose her mind when this mysterious change came over her.

Rosie Ledbetter had been, according to my mother's friends, as fine a woman as you'd ever want to know until she reached the "change," went haywire, and had to be sent to the asylum in Little Rock for three years. Even after she returned home, there was something terribly wrong with her that caused her to roam the town day and night and sometimes enter houses uninvited to sit in the living room until she was lured back outside once more.

Then there was Doctor Barton's widow who, at a certain time in her life, began barricading the doors of her house with dressers and tables and protecting herself further by wearing a winter coat even in hundred-degree weather. Since my mother knew that Lizzie Barton no longer used her stove for anything other than a place to set the slop jar, she feared Lizzie would starve without the casseroles she took her every week.

I accompanied my mother on these visits—she had no one to leave me with—so I stood with her on the porch listening to the scraping as Lizzie slowly pushed the furniture across the floor to free the door. The house we stepped into was like a cave, since all the shades were pulled, a cave full of the pervasive smell of garbage. Once we were inside the house, Lizzie scuttled to the far corner of the room, peering at us over her shoulder, a small woman huddled in a large coat with a wool cap pulled over her ears. She trusted Mother enough to let her into the house, but that was the extent of her social effort. I don't remember her ever saying a word to us.

"And that woman could play the piano better than anyone else in this town," Mother told me once as we climbed back in the car after our visit. "It breaks my heart to see her the way she is now."

There was one mad woman I never heard talked about when I was a child, perhaps because she died before I was born. I didn't know until I was grown that my own grandmother, my father's mother, was one of those who lost her mind at the change, going into a depression that refused to lift. One fine summer morning she got out of bed before anyone else in the house was awake, went to the kitchen, and drank some of the lye kept under the sink for making hominy. It took her a week to die.

After I left home and the small Arkansas town where I'd grown up, these stories fell into some deep recess of my mind, as many other things about my Arkansas childhood did. They seemed melodramatic, part of the Southern Gothic tradition that I learned about in literature classes. I was sure they had no bearing on my life.

Yet when I reached my late forties and knew I would be reaching menopause soon, the old stories about the horrors of the change of life did resurface in my mind from time to time as part of the vague dread I had about the prospect of menopause, a dread I hardly acknowledged since I thought it was irrational and unrealistic. I had read articles on menopause and knew that even if your hormones were thrown out of kilter at that time in your life, you could take estrogen pills and replace what was lost. And friends of mine who'd gone through menopause talked of it lightly. A writer I met at Yaddo, the artists' colony, said to me, "Mary, you'll sail through menopause as easily as I did. I didn't even have hot flashes. It was almost a nonevent."

If menopause could be a nonevent for my friend, I saw no reason why it shouldn't be one for me too. I told myself sharply there was no reason to dread it. After all, it would surely be convenient not to have to remember to pack Tampax when I traveled, not to concern myself with birth control any longer, to be free in a way I hadn't been since I was thirteen and started my first period. I dealt firmly with my dread and put it from my mind.

When I turned fifty, fifty-one with no change in the regularity of my monthly periods, I felt lulled. After all, it might be years before I entered menopause. Didn't women occasionally have babies when they were well into their fifties? I could continue exactly as I was for years and years.

But when I was fifty-two, I started a period that went on for three weeks. My family was renting a house on Okracoke Island, a short ferry ride from the tip of Cape Hatteras on the North Carolina Outer Banks, and I was constantly having to make trips to the one grocery store in the small town to buy Tampax.

I'd supposed that menopause would start with a skipped menstrual period or two, with a slackening. I hadn't expected it to begin instead with a flood. But I knew that the heavy bleeding was indicative of a change taking place in my body.

After the bleeding stopped, my periods continued for two months the same as usual. But on the third month, my period started late and was finished in a couple of days. And about this time I started waking in the night so hot I had to free myself from the blankets.

I had already decided that when I started menopause I would take estrogen replacement; I'm thin and fine boned, and I knew from my reading that fine boned women have a greater likelihood of developing osteoporosis in their old age.

When I visited my gynecologist, she agreed that I should take hormone replacement and prescribed a low dosage. My hot flashes, which had never been very troublesome anyway, ended. My periods grew scantier and scantier and finally stopped altogether. I knew then I had passed through menopause.

And, yes, it did seem almost a nonevent, with my life, so it seemed to me, the same as before. It was summer, and I spent the mornings as I usually did, writing in my study. In the afternoons I worked in my flowers, went for long bicycle rides alone or with friends, took the dogs for walks with my husband and daughter, who was spending the summer at home before going back to college.

The only problem was that I wasn't sleeping well, waking at two or three in the morning, unable to go back to sleep. But this had happened to me before. When I get overtired and my sleep rhythms are disturbed, or when something is worrying me, I go through a brief spell of sleeping badly. And something was worrying me that summer. My fifth novel had recently been published and though the reviews it had gotten had been mostly favorable, there hadn't been many of them, not as many as my previous novel had gotten. And since not many people knew of the novel's existence, sales had, of course, been few.

I knew there was a reason for this lack of attention that had nothing to do with the merits of the novel: The editor who had bought the manuscript and who had been enthusiastic about it left the publishing house while it was still in production—every writer's nightmare. But knowing there were reasons why this particular novel wasn't getting attention did almost nothing to ease my misery. My novel, into which I'd put so much passion and care, was dying, and I was unable to prevent its death. This seemed to me ample reason for my disturbed sleep.

That fall I taught fiction writing at Syracuse University, driving the five-hour round trip twice a week from our house near Lake Ontario, leaving home in the mornings at nine and returning at seven. The days were long, but I enjoyed the teaching. And through September and October, as the leaves turned orange and yellow and red, I even enjoyed the drive.

But I began the semester tired and became more tired as the weeks passed, since I was still waking in the early hours of the morning unable to go back to sleep again, still obsessing about my novel. I could see that the novel wouldn't make back its advance, and as a result of this it would be harder to sell my next novel; I could see a vicious circle being set in motion, one I could see no way of breaking. And the more I obsessed about the novel, the darker overtones the obsession took. It seemed to me that opportunities and possibilities were closing down; I would never have the kind of writing success I longed for, nor any other kind.

At two-thirty in the morning, when my eyes suddenly opened, I saw myself on a downward slide that would end only with my death. My life was closing down, or at least closing in. I was no longer young; I was starting to look middle aged. There were wrinkles in my skin, my jaw no longer quite firm. All of this became part of the murky soup of my obsessing. And I saw, in those early morning hours, that I had been very wrong to suppose menopause had been a nonevent in my life. On the contrary, it now seemed to me that menopause had opened the way to all the hope-lessness I was beginning to feel.

During the daylight hours, however, I seldom thought about the wor-ries that filled my nights. I prepared classes, taught, spent evenings with friends or went to a movie with my husband. My life seemed normal except for my increasing tiredness.

My teaching days were Mondays and Wednesdays, and on the drive home Wednesday evenings I felt relieved since I knew I would have four days without obligations, four days to try to get over my insomnia. Other bouts of sleeplessness I'd had before this had never lasted much longer than a week; after that my usual sleep rhythms reasserted themselves once more. So each night when I went to bed, I thought this might be the night I would sleep eight hours straight through without waking once, my insomnia releasing its hold.

But instead of easing, my insomnia grew worse. Before this, I'd had no trouble falling asleep; sleeplessness came later in the night. But as the fall continued into early November, something more disturbing hap-pened. Now I could not fall asleep at all. I simply stopped sleeping. When this happened, my other worries slipped into the background. My insom-nia became my chief source of concern.

I tried every trick I knew to get myself to relax: I tensed muscles and then released them again, starting with my toes and ending with my fore-head; I visualized a beautiful meadow full of summer wild flowers and imagined lying in the grass with the sun on my face; I drank warm milk and honey before I went to bed; I read, watched television. Nothing worked. I seemed to have forgotten how to sleep.

My doctor prescribed sleeping pills, and for a short time these seemed to help. At least when I took the pills I was able to sleep for a few hours. But the sleep I got when I took the pills wasn't restful. I woke after a few hours with the same numbing exhaustion I'd felt when I crawled into bed.

The drive to Syracuse and the effort required to teach my classes became an ordeal. During my office hours, between visits from students, I lay on the floor of my office feeling like a zombie, almost too exhausted to move.

My goal became simply to get through the semester until Thanksgiv-ing. I'd have nearly a week off then followed by only another two and a half weeks of classes. And after the semester ended I could stay in bed. For days, weeks, for the rest of my life. This was the only hope I held for myself—simply to lie in bed.

The week before Thanksgiving it snowed heavily. I drove to Syracuse at a crawl, for seconds at a time coming to a halt, unable to see anything except a swirling white outside the windows of the car. I reached my one o'clock literature class five minutes late and released my students early since I could see that the snow blowing against the classroom windows wasn't diminishing. I knew the New York Thruway could be closed at any time and this frightened me.

Though I knew I would be wise to spend that night in Syracuse, the thought of being unable to get home filled me with panic. I simply had to get back to my own bed.

And so I drove home in a strange state that had gone almost beyond exhaustion, my mind and body having seemingly parted company with one another, leaving my body to struggle on its own while my mind went off onto odd paths. In the snow driving into my headlights I saw faces; once a white animal leaped from one side of the road to the other.

When I got home my husband had dinner waiting, but I was past eating.

"I don't think I'll ever get over this," I told him as I made my way slowly up the stairs. "I'm not ever going to be able to sleep again."

"I'm taking you to the doctor tomorrow," he said, and I could hear the fear in his voice. "And I'm telephoning the English department and telling them you're sick. You can't meet your Wednesday class, and if you're not better after Thanksgiving, you can't go back then, either."

I took my shoes off and got into bed, doubting I would ever have the strength to get out of it again. I lay looking at the ceiling, listening to my husband feeding the cats in the kitchen, but everything I saw or heard seemed a great way off. I was in one place and the rest of the world in another, and though I felt a great longing to join the ordinary world again, the one where people slept without even thinking about it, where they sat at kitchen tables eating dinner with their families, laughing about something that had happened in the day, it seemed impossible that I would ever be able to join the world again.

Was this what it meant to lose your mind?

As tired as my brain was, this thought jolted it from its daze. I thought about those women from my childhood and wondered—had they gone through the kind of despair I'd felt for the last three months? Had the narrow boundaries of their world in a small, rural town diminished to a space that left them no breathing room, so their hopelessness drove them to escape in what must have seemed to them the only way open? By losing their hold on reality altogether?

I thought it was very possible they had felt this way and had taken a back door escape from one set of miseries to another. As I lay beside my sleeping husband, hearing the snow whispering against the windows, I felt I understood them as I never had before. I saw that those old stories from my childhood had been about more than oddity or colorful eccentricity. They were evidence of pain I hadn't paid attention to before.

I thought about my grandmother's slipping quietly from her bed one early summer morning when the birds were singing, sliding from a bed that had offered her no rest or peace, walking silently and purposefully to the kitchen, having planned her escape during the long hours of the night. I wondered if she had hesitated when she lifted the bottle of lye to her lips, but I didn't think she had. By the time she came to stand at the sink with the bottle in her hands, I felt sure she knew what she wanted to do.

When I imagined that early morning scene of nearly eighty years before, I felt close to my grandmother. But at the same time I knew that our circumstances were very different. I might feel that my life was closing down, that nothing good would ever happen to me again, but I had only to remember those women from my childhood to realize how little truth there was in those fears of mine.

Yes, it's difficult to give up the illusion of youth; it's never easy to accept that one is growing old. It would be a mistake to gloss over this very real pain as I had tried to do when I insisted to myself that menopause was a nonevent in my life, pretending it had no importance or significance.

But on that night when I reached my own point of greatest misery, I was also able to see that pain in perspective. I had far more opportunities than the women of my grandmother's generation had had. I was healthy (or had been before I stopped sleeping), energetic, and I wasn't finished as a writer. I had been, in fact, thinking about a new novel before I became too exhausted to work on it and though I had no guarantee any future novel of mine would be published, I wouldn't let that stop me from writing.

I felt I understood how those women from my past had reached such despair they saw no way out, but I wasn't one of them. I wasn't going to lose my mind. I wasn't going to die—not immediately, at least.

It would make a good ending of this story to say that I instantly fell into a deep sleep that was uninterrupted for ten hours, that I woke from that sleep refreshed and renewed, my insomnia and misery overcome. That, however, is not quite the way it was.

But after that night I was able to start getting back into the old rhythms and habits of sleep again, able to nap for an hour or two here, an hour or two there. Within two weeks I was sleeping through the night again. I felt I had been through a crisis and survived.

My life was not, of course, exactly the same as it had been before those months of insomnia or before menopause—I knew I would never be quite as concerned about aging or even about failure as I had been before I was forced to come to terms with them. I had come to see that if we don't accept change in our lives then we start to die, and I wasn't ready to do that just yet. Having passed through one change in my life, I was ready to move on to the next.

CATHERINE REID

Menopausal Eyebrows

The women at my bank look like transvestites. Or is it that the drag queens who come out after midnight look like the women at my bank? They do heels the same way. And hair; so much hair and nails. And lips that glisten in shades of red, though deciding if that's for pain or pleasure is like asking if this glass is half full or half empty, and we all know the answer is situation dependent.

Like menopause as a marker of some women's lives. If you're fifty, the "half" might be easier to place. But if you're thirty-eight it can be somewhat disorienting, especially if, like me, you're tall and thin and have started wearing your hair short again. On those days that I'm not in a skirt or a Woman's attire, people often mistake me for a boy, or they call me "Sir," which makes me cranky, that prickly restlessness under my skin that has settled in a lot lately, crabbiness that intends to stay even though I know how easily identity gets hauled on, *as easy as stockings, up, up, the light shimmery off that stretched-fine nylon, the urge tightening to saunter and invite; perhaps with a silk slip, a slinkier dress, a boa to flip and keep the crowds rowdy.*

If the women at my bank know that there are places in town where midnight becomes a kind of Cinderella Hour in reverse (instead of going to rags they've gone to excess), and where it's clothes, not anatomy, that defines the way to act—well, if they know, they don't let on. But that's typical of the daylight hours, when our imaginations tell us more than the people around us of their lives. It is in the dark that stories drive performance, and if sex is in the air and gender on the move, then anyone can see how all dress is drag and every part has its costume. With a little humor and some makeup, a good razor and sturdy corsets, almost anyone can pass as some Other.

Though only hormones will work on those sex-linked voices.

Which doesn't seem to be a problem for any of the women at my bank, so I view them as female impersonators. I don't know how they view me. They smile a lot and pass on messages if my partner isn't with me, and they seem at ease with how we share an account. Of course, they may also be thinking: *That darker one, she could be someone's Wife or Mother. But the bony one who travels with her? No way she's beginning menopause. Too young. Too boyish. Probably never dripped blood in the first place.*

That's the part that will never change, however, no matter whether we construct gender from the shoes up or the hairdo down. This is still the sex of me, and this the sudden body-rage of sweat and nastiness that's here and gone again, as fast as a summer thunderstorm.

My grandmother was thirty-eight when she went into menopause; so was my mother, though she had planned to have another six kids. Neither of them was ever called "Sir" or mistaken for her husband's daughter, but I was carded a few weeks ago at the local supermarket when I added a six-pack of beer to the week's groceries (luckily, the young whippersnapper didn't stop me when I was in one of *those* moods). And it took me several days before I could again savor this new link, *in the female way,* with the women in my family, a bridge for the *lesbian!* and *no-children!* gaps. Though these family members may not have the genes to enjoy a queen in her finery or a baby dyke in her bad boots and leather, still they are a part of me. In fact, *they helped make me this way.* But that is another story.

What I know of this story and of being thirty-eight is that it looks more like a beginning than a halfway place (especially since my grandmother is ninety and still holding her own). I also know that thirty-eight is a woman's *sexual prime,* and though I continue to be the one with more energy and appetite, I realize that could change real soon.

My partner and I joke about who will be pushing whose wheelchair, but mostly, I don't want to become more brittle or dry. There is already too much stiffness in my WASP-culture and skin, a wrinkle-lipped prim that would be making even deeper grooves if I hadn't seen the gender outlaws' parodies. They keep me from taking this too seriously. So does my partner, who sees me looking weepy or wanting to crawl into her lap and says, *You can't be starting menopause, you're barely out of puberty.*

It's true, my eyes do leak a lot, and my hands will probably shake even more as the years go by. My bones will probably break first, too, though my lover has seven years on me and far more silver in her hair. We'll miss the drama of going through *the Change* at the same time (she'll be buying Tampax for another ten years, easy), but I'll have a reason to smile the next time a young salesclerk sees the two of us together and begins to suspect *that dark one, she could be the Mother,* because hormonally I am the oldest one, *and surely that means I am the wisest.*

In the long run, though, neither of us will feel much more than *At last!* said with much relief. And *Ahhh.* For the matter, I doubt many lesbians will be too alarmed about all this aging—which is not to say there won't be aching and worry (over sleep and libido and constipation, especially when those night sweats insist everything else STOP; or when our cynicism rises up over those well-touted mainstream remedies—ERT—that have never been too kind to women). Most of us have already faced the mirror and figured out that this package we've been given is not of the average. We're used to being different, the odd one out, the exception to the rule. So why should experiencing gray and wrinkly, or a strangely dry vagina, be other than another kind of adventure? *(But please, not the hump! Not that dowager's hump!)* Besides, now that lesbians can have kids, if and when we want to get pregnant (even if our bleeding has stopped!), menopause doesn't need to mean anything has ended (well, maybe some of that interest in sex).

As lesbians, we've survived insult and exclusion, harassment and despair, so readying for this next step is like preparing for a long trip when we know some of the variables ahead of time. There's a food box that needs to be packed, with lots of tofu and yams (rumor has it they act like estrogen); and of course a trunk to be filled with a wide assortment of clothes (add a few kinds of pads, perhaps some extra *Attends*); and then make room for the medicine kit, which might have some KY Jelly and a tube of estrogen cream in addition to all those bottles of calcium. Maybe someone will even stick a scented note in the lingerie: *Remember to do your exercises. Remember to come home to me.*

Despite all this careful planning, though, I can't quite stop wondering where all the blood is going to go. Not the monthly period blood, because I'll be glad when the last trace is finally gone, but the blood that has been in my poems and dreams; the raw monthly smell that buoyed me and clung to me, though no one ever seemed to turn toward it, *Where have you been? What have you been eating?* It just seemed to be a cloud I lived in on those days, thinking, *earth, sweat, sex;* feeling that bodily brew of belly-soft and fierce, too.

I also wonder if I will have enough stored rhythm, now that I don't live near the sea or have a moon visible every night from the windows. I believe Judy Grahn's theory, that by watching when they bled and how it seemed to happen with the moon, early women invented time as well as consciousness. I'm not sure what she says about menopausal women, but I sure hope I maintain the sense of cycles. I like to imagine the feelings are ingrained, the way my body still craves the first spring greens (coltsfoot and violets, fiddleheads and asparagus), even though I live now in the South, where there's garden greenery year round. Or the way my body continues to rock whenever we return from hours or days at the ocean, back and forth with the waves, up and down. In my fantasy, however, these rhythms will come from much deeper and will ripple through us far longer.

When they first look at me, the women at my bank might never believe that I really am in touch with my femme side. A few years ago it came to me, lying in bed after another back injury: *I don't have to be butch any more.* Of course, it helped that this strong femme had entered my life and was baking cookies for me at the time. And since she could butch when she needed to—and owned a chainsaw and a Cuisinart and a house in the woods—pretty soon we began swapping roles. Right off, I found I liked it. *A little hairspray to hold these new upsweeps. Some mascara to show off these lashes. And that sexy surprise of smooth skin and sheer hose.*

Clearly butch had too much hurt attached (something you're not supposed to notice except when a sympathetic femme is around) and it meant too many roof peaks with tight ropes and steep ladders, and narrow crawl spaces under houses or cars, with oil stains that just wouldn't come out. . . .

Femme is much easier and so much gentler on the flesh, though there are still those moments, like in those fluorescent-lit dressing rooms. *Is this what we really wear? Is this the way we're supposed to look?* But femme also meant a chance for long hair, which I wore twisted up in back. And occasionally a bra to display what I had in front. And I really didn't have to shorten my stride. *All those double takes, when I travel across campus in boots and long skirts; all those young men scurrying to open doors for me.* Femme means that on certain days I let the bagboy carry out my groceries. I take my car to SuperLube and pay someone else to do the dirty work. And since we live now in this easy-to-tend house, it's a simple wrist action with this little unit on the wall whenever I'm too cold or too hot.

But then I cut my hair, very quick, very short, and when I'm in jeans and a T-shirt, no one opens the door for me, and those double takes when the two of us travel together are to see if maybe I am her son. Which means it's clear once again how little estrogen and gender have to do with one another. And how it's in my sex that I feel it, in my womb and in my thighs.

"It affects the thighs chiefly," Virginia Woolf wrote in her diary. "And I want to burst into tears, but have nothing to cry for. . . . Partly T. of L. I wonder? A physical feeling as if I were drumming slightly in the veins: very cold: impotent: and terrified. As if I were exposed on a high ledge in full light" (March 1, 1937).

A slight drumming, a noise in my brain; a whirl that keeps away whatever isn't happening inside me. I think. Though it may be more mental than hormonal; "T of L" may mean listening to whatever I want to, and seeing only that which holds my interest.

I know I'm already more honest, which might have to do with what's happening to my eyebrows. No one hinted that this could be where the best change was going to take place. But there they are, a few of them erratically long, curling up my forehead some mornings, other times caught in my lashes. Perhaps I will mascara them, too, so they'll show from a distance, pointing out the ways our bodies do this. The way we can be more reckless if we want to, and definitely more suspect and ornery.

The way ours is the only yard of ferns and wildflowers; we don't do lawnmowers or loud leafblowers or clothesdryers that churn in the garage, preferring the sounds of treefrogs and crickets and owls. And we would rather see eyebrow hairs like these, that start bushing out like vines, because then this crabbiness makes sense. *It's her Time of Life,* they'll say; or, *She's having the Time of her Life,* and they'll quit getting stumped by my age or asking for ID at the checkout. They'll just wave me right on through because it's clear from those hairs that they don't want me to linger, that there's no telling what else I might do.

And maybe when this is all over, I'll finally be a bit smarter (and without, of course, the weight of *that hump*). I know I'll be smiling when the queens go sashaying because this is one part that they'll never do. And I expect there to be days when the women at my bank will look at me and understand just how I'm being. I might even surprise them and go in sometime with high hair or luscious new nail color. But I doubt that I'll ever stop this other odd wondering, *Will nose hairs come next? Will long chin hairs?*

DENISE SPITZER

More than the Change:
Diversity and Flexibility
in Menopausal Experience

⌖

By the year 2000, over 700 million women worldwide will be experiencing or will have passed through menopause (Diczfalusy 1986). These women come from various cultural and socioeconomic backgrounds; they possess differing values and have different access to resources—and their experiences of menopause vary.

Sociocultural Diversity and Menopause

How does menopause differ cross-culturally? To explore these differences, we must look at the meanings of menopause, the view of aging and of mid-life, the status of women, the beliefs and values people share and the roles women may take on in various cultures. Research shows that women's experience of menopause is extremely diverse (Spitzer 1994). Perhaps the most common feature of menopause found cross-culturally is role change. Role changes are shifts in the expected or anticipated activities or responsibilities of women. What this means is that in numerous cultures, postmenopausal women can take on new roles that had previously been denied them. Women can become elders or wise women as in Burkina Faso (Diop 1989); healers or midwives; they can take on religious roles; or, like !Kung women of southern Africa, they can be at the peak of their spiritual power (Shostak 1981). Female traders in West Africa can expand their roles as postmenopausal women are no longer deemed a sexual threat and are able to venture farther afield (Coles 1991; Henderson 1969).

Postmenopause, however, is not a period of wellness and respect for all non-Western women. For example, changes in roles at menopause are not universally positive; Twi and Zulu women may lose status because they can no longer bear children. As a result, their husbands may remarry and shift their attention to younger and potentially fertile wives (Berglund 1976; Field 1960). This loss of childbearing potential may be particularly difficult for women who are focused primarily on parenting; however, in some cultures, women have the ability to extend this role through adoption or grandmothering.

If we take a closer look at the changes in role and status of women at middle age, we see that many of these role shifts do not actually occur at menopause. Other social events such as the marriage of the eldest child or birth of a grandchild might herald a change in women's status at times other than menopause. Hausa women in Nigeria, for instance, may simply adopt a postmenopausal role when it suits them; they may move away from their husbands, expand their trading networks, re-marry if they are divorced, select mates for their children, or adopt more children by claiming status as a middle-aged woman—a label generally applied to postmenopausal women up to about age sixty (Coles 1991).

In other cases where women are able to take on more positive postmenopausal roles or increased prestige, not all members of a culture are able to experience these improvements in status. For Muslim women in the Sudan, for example, postmenopause is a time of increased freedom, a chance for them to become the head of a genealogical line, to arrange marriages and to speak out in public, but only if they are married. Women who are divorced, widowed or deemed too old to re-marry actually experience a decline in status in middle age (Boddy 1985).

Women's ability to access positive postmenopausal roles is also changing due to global economic pressures. For example, the power base of Tswana women in Botswana is traditionally centered in the extended family household. Women expect to experience increased prestige at middle age as they take on more responsibility as household managers and bearers of tradition to pass on to their grandchildren. But that power base is fast eroding as sons are compelled to move away in order to find work in more prosperous locations (Suggs 1986). A similar situation seems to be occurring in Turkey, where middle-aged women could traditionally anticipate receiving increased prestige as well as household assistance from members of their extended family as they matured. However, more and more family members are moving to urban areas, leaving mature women without the anticipated support of their families (Delaney 1988).

Cultural diversity in menopausal experiences is also related to women's attitudes toward menstruation. Although we might expect that negative attitudes toward menstruation would translate into positive attitudes toward menopause, this does not appear to follow (Spitzer 1994). When menstrual blood is seen as polluting or dirty, menstruation itself may be considered beneficial, as the offending menstrual blood is eliminated from the body. For women in some cultures, menopause is viewed as the retention of menstrual blood; the accumulation of menstrual blood then is believed to cause any number of complaints including headaches, hot flashes and the accumulation of toxins. Even in a single community, attitudes toward menstruation and menopause can be diametrically opposed. Skultans's (1970) study in a Welsh village, for example, revealed that some women felt that menstruation was a symbol of fertility and heavy menstrual bleeding was beneficial. These women were generally satisfied with their lives in terms defined by their families and village life; for them, menopause posed a threat to their femininity. Single and childless women in the community, however, were more likely to believe that they should avoid blood loss at menstruation; for these women, menopause was not a troubling prospect.

Some people claim that non-Western women generally experience positive changes after menopause. These claims are often based on the idea that women in many cultures are released from menstrual taboos and that this must be beneficial. In this regard, women who practice menstrual taboos, which regulate the behavior of menstruating women through physical separation from others or prohibitions regarding certain daily activities, are considered superstitious and primitive. Release from these prohibitions, it is reasoned, must be a cause for celebration. Yet, in many instances women who practice menstrual taboos or regulations see menstruation as a positive phenomenon. Among Yurok Indians of California, for example, menstrual separation allows women to pursue spiritual activities and releases them from mundane obligations (Buckley 1993); Tamil women have complained to one researcher that their workload increases after menopause because they no longer have a monthly period of rest (Reynolds 1987). Traditional Navajo women, who adhere to numerous taboos during menstruation such as refraining from touching children or livestock or visiting the ill, regard menstruation as cleansing; therefore, its loss may be detrimental to a woman's health (Wright 1982). In New Zealand, Maori women spend time together during menstruation, a practice that has the effect of increasing female solidarity and support throughout their lives (Sinclair 1985).

Women's attitudes toward menopause itself are also associated with the cultural construction of menopause. By the cultural construction of

menopause, I mean the set of symptoms or behaviors that are attributed
to menopause by members of a cultural grouping. The cultural construction of menopause differs widely. For instance, Indian women resid-
ing near Delhi have reported that the menopausal transition is of little
consequence to them, although many were pleased to have both their
menstrual cycle and childbearing over. These women did report experiencing hot flashes; however, they were considered to be a part of aging
rather then attributable to menopause (Vatuk 1975).

The cultural construction of menopause provides the backdrop
for stereotypes of the menopausal woman that change not only cross-
culturally, but also over time. In North America, for example, the symptoms of menopause now include osteoporosis and vaginal atrophy,
whereas formerly involutional melancholia, a form of depression believed
to occur at menopause, and digestive problems were the predominant
symptoms (Mittness 1983). During the Victorian age, menopausal symptoms included hysteria, headaches, nervous depression and even insanity
(Penrose 1900). Weakening eyesight is considered a symptom of menopause by South Asian women (George 1985; Vatuk 1975). In Japan, sore
shoulders, tingling sensations, irritability and chills are most closely associated with *konneki*, or the menopausal transition, which is also regarded
as lasting almost seven years (Lock, Kaufert and Gilbert 1988; Rosenberger 1986)—in contrast with the medical construction of menopause,
which defines it as lasting two years, one year prior to and one year after
the last menstrual cycle.

Cultural expectations of menopause, in terms of anticipated complaints or role changes, shape the manner in which a woman responds to
the menopausal transition. A number of studies carried out in the West
demonstrate a link between attitudes toward menopause and the rate of
menopausal complaints. We also find that symptoms regarded as troublesome in some cultures may be perceived as valuable in others. Hot
flashes, for example, can be perceived as cleansing the body; women in
rural Newfoundland believe that hot flashes help in reducing hyper-
tension and speeding up the pace of the menopausal transition (Davis
1983), and Mexican-American women report that they are important
in cleansing the body of accumulated menstrual blood (Kay 1982).

If we look at a broader picture, we find that women's menopausal
experiences are also related to economic development. Women in industrialized countries are faced with a decline of socially recognized prestigious postmenopausal roles; they tend to report more physical and
psychological complaints than women in lesser industrialized coun-

tries.* However, women who live in urban areas of industrializing nations such as Nigeria, Thailand and Indonesia appear to conform to this pattern of fewer prestigious roles and more complaints. This contrasts with the pattern of responses to menopause found in rural areas of these industrializing countries, as well as industrialized nations such as Greece and Portugal. In these areas, culturally prestigious postmenopausal roles for women were commonly found, accompanied by positive attitudes toward menopause.

A woman's social situation can also affect her menopausal experiences. Studies done in the West show that stress appears to have a large impact on menopausal symptoms. One British study found that women who were depressed after menopause suffered from sleep disorders and were likely to be coping with a number of stressful life events including possible illness and were less inclined to exercise (Hunter 1992). In a summary of European surveys conducted on menopause, Greene (1990) found that women with lower incomes, less job satisfaction, a reduced social network and low levels of education were more likely to experience menopause as stressful.

Class differences in menopausal complaints have been recorded in a number of studies. Employed upper-class women appear to have fewer complaints than low income women, many of whom have fewer resources for coping and are in generally poorer health (Severne 1982). Class also has an obvious influence on the availability of health care choices.

PHYSIOLOGICAL DIVERSITY AND MENOPAUSE

Menopause does differ cross-culturally; however, menopause is still a biological phenomenon. The term "menopause" is defined by the World Health Organization as "the permanent cessation of menstruation resulting from the loss of ovarian function" (1980:8). From a medical per-

---

* I undertook a survey of the literature on menopause in ninety-six cultures to gain an understanding of the variables that have an impact on women's experience of menopause and to determine if there were any discernible trends in the data. Changes in subsistence activities from hunting-gathering, horticulture and agriculture to industrialization and increasing urbanization appeared to create conditions that were correlated to one particular trend found in industrialized and industrializing countries. Data from rural areas, where more traditional means of subsistence and community life persist, were correlated to another pattern. For a more detailed discussion of these findings see Spitzer 1994.

spective, menopausal status is generally determined retrospectively, following a six- to twelve-month absence of menstruation.

As women age, ova are depleted through the menstrual cycle until a critical number remain, triggering the end of menstruation. Menopause generally occurs at age fifty; however, malnourished populations are known to have an earlier average age at the onset (Ginsburg 1991). Ovaries undergo a number of changes during menopause, although they are still capable of producing estrogens; however, the main sites of estrogen production in postmenopausal women are in fat tissue, bone, hair follicles, liver, kidney and brain tissue (MacDonald 1979). Thus postmenopausal women are still capable of producing estrogen, but the sites of this production change and overall levels decline. As a result, estrogen levels in postmenopausal women vary considerably. Significantly, the presence or absence of the two most universal symptoms of menopause, hot flashes and vaginal dryness, is attributable to decreased but varying levels of estrogens.

Estrogen levels can change for a number of reasons; for instance, diet can have a significant impact on a woman's hormone levels. Changing from an omnivorous to a vegetarian diet over a two-month period, for example, has been shown to change the length of a woman's menstrual cycle (Hill, et al. 1977). Also the lack of hot flashes among Japanese menopausal women has led to a number of studies on the impact of diet on menopausal symptoms. Researchers have discovered that soy products such as tofu and miso contain plant estrogens that become biologically active when eaten (Aldercreutz, et al. 1991).

But diet is not the only influence on estrogen levels and consequently menopausal symptoms. Exercise, obesity, alcohol consumption, stress and sexual activity all have an impact on the physiological expression of menopause. Exercise increases beta-endorphins, which not only reduce pain sensation, but may be directly linked to hot flashes. Studies show that reduced levels of beta-endorphins may trigger the body's heat loss mechanism resulting in a hot flash (Casper and Yen 1985; Gannon 1988). As fat tissue is the major site of estrogen production in postmenopause, women who retain some body fat routinely have fewer menopausal complaints than slender women (see Campagnoli 1981 and Smith 1987). Alcohol consumption has also been found to increase estrogen levels sufficiently to reduce menopausal symptoms (Gavaler and Thiel 1992). On the other hand, stress can adversely affect menopausal symptoms as it results in decreased estrogen levels (Ballinger 1990). Sexual stimulation increases estrogen levels and appears to reduce hot flashes and vaginal dryness (Golub 1992).

EXPLANATORY MODELS AND MENOPAUSE
Given the great sociocultural and biological diversity associated with menopause, several questions remain. How are our ideas about menopause shaped? Do these ideas reflect the diversity of women's experience and do they serve menopausal women adequately? The literature on menopause is based on four competing, but by no means mutually exclusive, explanatory models used by both laypeople and professionals: medical, sociocultural, psychological and self-help. These models provide professionals and laypeople with an explanation of menopause that accounts for the cause of any problem, what outcomes a person can expect, what is perceived as appropriate treatment and what meaning, if any, is attached to the phenomenon (Kleinman 1980). Although popular understandings of a phenomenon may vary, these explanations generally differ from those of professionals. Often explanatory models voiced by professionals or experts take on the semblance of irrefutable truth. For instance, women who seek medical assistance during menopause learn biomedical vocabulary and explanations provided by their physicians; these professional explanations soon displace their own interpretations and experience (Dickson 1990). We need to see how these models address the diverse experiences of menopausal women.

THE MEDICAL MODEL
The medical model defines menopause as an endocrine deficiency disease similar to diabetes; thus menopause is regarded as a pathology that requires medical intervention. In the medical literature, menopausal women are often portrayed not just as aging, but decaying—menopausal women have *senile* vaginitis, *senescent* ovaries and vaginal *atrophy*. Subject to violent mood swings and incapable of making decisions, menopausal women are described as possessing scaling skin, flabby breasts and thickening waistlines (Logothetis 1991). A pharmaceutical company's brochure informs women that "you may experience tingling, and other skin sensations such as wrinkling skin . . . and a slight loss of bladder control" (Upjohn Company n.d.:3). Women's bodies are seen as both withering and out of control.

Treatment for menopause as an endocrine disorder comes in the form of hormone replacement therapy (HRT), which is reputed to reduce hot flashes, diminish bone loss and reduce the risk of heart disease. As sleep

loss due to night sweats is targeted as the cause of numerous psychological problems associated with menopause, HRT is recommended to resolve
these problems (Koeske 1982). Articles in the medical literature encourage physicians to start women on a course of HRT as soon as menopause
approaches and maintain treatment for up to ten years; if women are resistant, one physician (Ettinger 1988) suggest that his colleagues remind their
patients that living without estrogen is not natural; therefore, they are only
restoring their bodies to their natural state. Within the profit driven health
care industry, this appeal to the "natural" results in enormous profits for
the manufacturers of synthetic estrogen; Ayerst corporation earned over
$70 million in profits from synthetic estrogens in the 1970s, even before
HRT climbed in popularity (Dickson 1989).

Thus the medical model reinforces the medicalization of menopause,
encouraging the use of health care services and treatment. Medicalization
places control over women's bodies in the hands of professionals, endow-
ing them with the power to diagnose and to label menopause as a disease
and an abnormality. Furthermore, medicalization is not limited to Western countries; in Japan physicians view menopause as a disease of luxury
and claim that symptoms are due to a lack of outside interests or the
rejection of a nurturing role (Lock, Kaufert and Gilbert 1988). Japanese
physicians are now able to charge for services provided to women diagnosed with menopausal syndrome (Lock 1988).

Medical perspectives of menopause focus solely on the physiological:
female reproductive organs and sex hormones. There is little reference to
the personal or social factors that have an impact on women's complaints.
Furthermore, the medical model is based primarily on anecdotal information obtained from women who have already sought medical treatment, and these women may be experiencing greater difficulties than the
entire group of menopausal women in the population.

THE SOCIOCULTURAL MODEL

The sociocultural model of menopause, which makes reference to menopause as a cultural phenomenon, was developed by social scientists and is
sometimes quoted in the popular press to refute medical perspectives.
Although the cultural context of women's menopausal experiences is acknowledged in this model, menopausal complaints are regarded solely as
a Western phenomenon attributable to the low status of aging women
and a lack of socially recognized postmenopausal roles in Western societies. Thus, physician and anthropologist Wilbush (1980:58) writes that
"women in non-Western cultures do not recognize a critical time and are

not subject to any significant disturbance at the cessation of menses." Others suggest that increased status of non-Western women obtained through postive postmenopausal roles results in better mental health and accounts for reported differences in symptom expression (c.f. Bart 1969).

Numerous proponents of this model downplay the physiological changes that occur at menopause. Menopausal symptoms are tacitly regarded as not only culturally constructed, but psychological in nature, hence feeling good about aging is associated with an absence of menopausal complaints.

THE VULNERABILITY MODEL

The vulnerability model views menopause from a psychological perspective. According to its major proponent, Green (1984:134), "Adverse reaction shown by women during the climacteric is associated with pre-existing problems—psychological, social, marital, sexual, psychiatric—and that these reactions are in turn mediated by pre-existing psychosocial and socio-demographic factors, more so than by factors thought to be peculiar to, or occurring particularly at that time." Essentially, this model views distress at menopause as the straw that breaks the camel's back. Menopause itself may not be a stressful or troublesome phenomenon, but if it is accompanied by numerous stressful life events, this might affect a woman's ability to cope with the transition.

Thus far the vulnerability model has only been applied to Western studies and has not been proven to be applicable cross-culturally. Some of the social pressures associated with middle age identified in the model are not universal; role changes do not necessarily occur at menopause and therefore cannot be responsible for a reaction in coping ability. Furthermore, this model tends to overlook the biological aspects of menopause and relates the suffering that some women experience to their inability to cope, thus belittling rather than legitimating their experiences.

THE SELF-HELP MODEL

Self-help and other popular explanatory models of menopause found in the West represent the efforts of women to gain greater control over the sharing of information regarding menopause and over their bodies. These models often use the sociocultural model as a critique of other explanatory models and advocate self-help and alternative healing modalities as a method of coping with menopausal symptoms. Some popular writers endorse the use of HRT, perhaps with greater caution than medical model advocates, while other authors suggest women try herbal remedies and alternative therapies to alleviate symptoms.

Generally, women are encouraged to talk about menopause with each other and in public. No longer confined to the feminist press or women's magazines, menopause has become a subject for newspapers and television. Women are encouraged to celebrate menopause; it is "an opportunity for long-delayed self-indulgence and reflection: a chance to reassess priorities and focus creative energies in new directions, a time to travel or concentrate on interests put on hold during child rearing" (Barsky 1992:52). Women's desire for greater control over their menopausal experiences has created new outlets for sharing information through self-help groups, newsletters, public forums and electronic discussion groups. This new wealth of information sharing is not devoid of advice: Much of the literature concentrates on self-care for women rather than on symptoms (McElmurray and Huddleston 1991). Women are encouraged to maintain balance in their lives, to eat a healthy diet, to oil their skin and to join menopause support groups (Kaufert 1982). Some advisors suggest that women endow menopause with their own meaning through creating their own rites of passage or reclaiming their right to be visible as middle-aged women in a society that attends only to youth (Greer 1991).

Self-help approaches are valuable to certain sectors of the population; however, they are infused with the notions of individualism and self-care; notions that are both culture- and class-bound. A woman requires adequate financial and personal resources in order to eat well, pamper herself or attend a support group. These are luxuries that may be out of reach for lower income women, and their needs are often overlooked in the literature.

THE DIVERSITY OF MENOPAUSAL EXPERIENCE AND EXPERT ADVICE

Thus menopause is a disease, a cultural phenomenon without reference to biology, an indicator of stress or a time for self and celebration. The difficulty with these explanatory models is that each projects an image of the stereotypical menopausal woman, a measuring stick to which women can be compared or can compare themselves. The resulting stereotypes of menopausal women lend themselves to the daunting amount of literature on menopause that is replicated in the popular media. According to the medical model, she is depressed, sweaty, eager to maintain sexual attraction and requires HRT, the panacea for all menopausal women; refusal to comply is a threat to her sexual well-being or bone health.

Advocates of the sociocultural and self-help models suggest that Western women can be jubilant, asexual and symptom-free only if they are pleased to have reached this phase of their lives, like all non-Western women.

Although menopause is a universal female biological phenomenon, it is also a product of personal, environmental and cultural factors that interact at all levels and exist in political, economic and historical context—factors not taken into account in the dominant explanatory models. Normative explanations of menopause are based on the assumption that all members of a group are a collection of similar bodies who will incorporate identical information from their cultural and physical environments and react in a similar fashion. When attempts are made to describe an average and a range of experience, quite often the description of the average becomes the focus that develops into the stereotype of a modal individual that resembles no one. Thus, normative models perpetuate the myth of the average menopausal woman, an image with which other women may compare themselves and not find themselves reflected; this discrepancy between stereotype and individual experience can become a source of anxiety for women. Most importantly, normative models and the versions of truth that accompany them are cut off from women's life experiences and voice.

In eighteenth-century Europe, the interior of the body was visualized as a miasma: fluid and shifting, bound by the semi-porous confines of the skin (Duden 1991). Within the next century, the body, placed under scrutiny of the medical gaze, solidified. Like the inner workings of a clock, the elements of the body were laid bare, defined and composed in a logical and predictable order. This concept of the body, represented by translucent life-size plastic models in the student anatomy lab, is one in which cause and effect are readily observed. It is a body that exists alone, the product of the internal functioning of its discrete parts. This image of the isolated, uniform and predictable body has allowed for the ongoing production of medical knowledge and advice—advice that is assumed to be universally applicable.

The normative aspect to all of the explanatory models is based on this uniformity, just like an assembly line. The body as product and as machine become identical in nature. However, the body is far more flexible and its working more elusive than the lifeless model hanging in the anatomy lab would suggest. On a daily basis the body shifts, adjusts and compensates; rather than remaining static, we change.

It is this flexibility of our bodies and personal response to the environment that has not been adequately accounted for in the menopausal literature. Expert advice may be useful when referring to the repair of electrical devices, but it does not address the diverse realities of women's experience, realities that reflect the variability and flexibility of women themselves. Although women need information, both to understand the biological basis of menopause and to become aware of and share in the experiences of others, the primary focus for women should consist of the shaping of their own menopausal transition.

WORKS CITED

Aldercreutz, Hermann, Hideo Honjo, Akane Higashi, Theodore Fotsis, Esa Hämäläinen, Takeshi Hasegawa and Hiroji Okada
   1991 Urinary Excretion of Lignans and Isoflavanoid Phytoestrogens in Japanese Men and Women Consuming a Traditional Japanese Diet. *American Journal of Clinical Nutrition* 54:1087–1092.

Ballinger, Susan
   1985 Psychosocial Stress and Symptoms of Menopause: A Comparative Study of Menopause Clinic Patients and Non-Patients. *Maturitas* 7: 315–327.
   1990 Stresses as a Factor in Lowered Estrogen Levels in Early Post-menopause. *Annals of the New York Academy of Sciences* 592 (June 13): 95–113.

Barsky, Lesley
   1992 Ready, Set, Manage Your Menopause! *Chatelaine* February 50–52, 82–84.

Bart, Pauline
   1969 Why Women's Status Changes in Middle Age: The Turn of the Social Ferris Wheel. *Sociological Symposium* 3:1–18.

Berglund, Alex-Ivar
   1976 *Zulu Thought—Patterns and Symbolism*. Uppsala: Institute of Missionary Research.

Boddy, Janice
   1985 Bucking the Agnatic System: Status and Strategies in Rural Northern Sudan. In *In Her Prime: A New View of Middle-Aged Women*, Judith Brown and Virginia Kerns, eds. South Hadley: Bergin and Garvey Publishers.

Buckley, Thomas
   1993 Menstruation and the Power of Yurok Women. In *Gender in Cross-Cultural Perspective*, Caroline B. Brettel and Carolyn F. Sargent, eds. Berkeley: University of California Press.

Campagnoli, C., G. Morra, P. Belforte, L. Belforte and L. Prelat Tonsijin
   1981 Climacteric Symptoms According to Body-Weight in Women of Different Socio-Economic Groups. *Maturitad* 3:279–287.

Casper, R. F. and S. S. C. Yen
   1985 Neuroendocrinology of Menopausal Hot Flushes: An Hypothesis of the Flush Mechanism. *Clinical Endocrinology* 22:293–312.

Coles, Catherine
    1991 Hausa Society: Power and Authority in Urban Nigeria. In *Anthropology 90/91*, Elvio Angeloni, ed. Guilford, Conn.: Dushkin.

Davis, Dona Lee
    1983 *Blood and Nerves: An Ethnographic Focus on Menopause.* St. John's: Institute of Social and Economic Research, Memorial University of Newfoundland.

Delaney, Carol
    1988 Mortal Flow: Menstruation in Turkish Village Society. In *Blood Magic: The Anthropology of Menstruation*, Thomas Buckley and Alma Gottlieb, eds. Berkeley: University of California Press.

Dickson, Geri L.
    1989 *The Knowledge of Menopause: An Analysis of Scientific and Everyday Discourses.* Unpublished Ph.D. dissertation, University of Wisconsin-Madison.
    1990 A Feminist Post-Structuralist Analysis of the Knowledge of Menopause. *Advances in Nursing Science* 12(3) Apr.: 15–31.

Diczfalusy, Egon
    1986 Menopause, Developing Countries and the 21st Century. *Acta Obstetrics and Gynecology Scandinavian Supplement* 134:45–57.

Diop, Amadou Moustapha
    1989 The Place of the Elderly in African Society. *Impact of Science on Society* 153:93-98.

Duden, Barbara
    1991 *The Woman Beneath the Skin: A Doctor's Patients in 18th Century Germany.* Cambridge: Harvard University Press.

Ettinger, Bruce
    1988 Optimal Use of Postmenopausal Hormone Replacement. *Obstetrics and Gynecology* (Supplement) 72(5): 31–36.

Field, Margaret Joyce
    1960 *Search for Security: An Ethnographic Study of Rural Ghana.* Evanston, Ill.: Northwestern University Press.

Gannon, Linda
    1988 The Potential Role of Exercise in the Alleviation of Menstrual Disorders and Menopausal Symptoms: A Theoretical Synthesis of Recent Research. *Women and Health* 14(2): 105–127.

Gavaler, Judith S. and David H. Van Thiel
    1992 The Association Between Moderate Alcoholic Beverage Consump-

tion and Serum Estradiol and Testosterone Levels in Normal Post-menopausal Women: Relationship to the Literature. *Alcoholism: Clinical and Experimental Research* 16(1): 87–92.

George, Theresa
1985 *There is a Time for Everything: A Study of Menopausal/Climacteric Experience of Sikh Women in Canada.* Unpublished Ph.D. dissertation, University of Utah.

Ginsburg, Jean
1991 What Determines the Age at the Menopause? *British Medical Journal* 302:1288–1289.

Golub, Sharon
1992 *Periods: From Menarche to Menopause.* Newbury Park: Sage Publications.

Greene, John C.
1984 *The Social and Psychological Origins of the Climacteric Syndrome.* Hants, Gower Publishing Co., Ltd.
1990 Psychological Influences and Life Events at the Time of Menopause. In *The Meanings of Menopause: Historical, Medical and Clinical Perspectives*, Ruth Formek, ed. Hillsdale: The Analytic Press.

Greer, Germaine
1991 *The Change: Women, Aging and the Menopause.* Toronto: Alfred A. Knopf Canada.

Hill, Peter, P. Chan, L. Cohen, E. Wynder and K. Kuno
1977 Diet and Endocrine Related Cancer. *Cancer* 39:1820–1826.

Hunter, Myra
1992 The South-East England Longitudinal Study of the Climacteric and Post-Menopause. *Maturitas* 14:117–126.

Kaufert, Patricia
1982 Myth and the Menopause. *Sociology of Health and Illness* 4(2): 141–166.

Kay, Margarita, Ann Voda, Guadelupe Olivas, Frances Ries and Margaret Imle
1982 Ethnography of the Menopause-Related Hot Flash. *Maturitas* 4:217–227.

Kleinman, Arthur
1980 *Patients and Healers in the Context of Culture.* Berkeley: University of California Press.

Koeske, Randi Daimon
  1982 Toward a Biosocial Paradigm for Menopause Research: Lessons and Contributions from Behavioural Sciences. In *Changing Perspectives on Menopause*, Ann Voda, Myra Dinnerstein and Sheryl O'Donnell, eds. Austin: University of Texas.

Lock, Margaret
  1988 New Japanese Mythologies: Faltering Discipline and the Ailing Housewife. *American Ethnologist* 15(1):43–61.

Lock, Margaret, Patricia Kaufert and Penny Gilbert
  1988 Cultural Construction of the Menopausal Syndrome: The Japanese Case. *Maturitas* 10:317–322.

Logothetis, Mary Lou
  1991 Our Legacy: Medical Views of the Menopausal Woman. In *Women of the 14th Moon: Writings on Menopause*, Dena Taylor and Amber Coverdale Sumrall, eds. Freedom: The Crossing Press.

MacDonald, P. C.
  1979 Determinants of the Rate of Estrogen Formation in Postmenopausal Women. *European Journal of Obstetrics, Gynecology and Reproductive Biology* 9(3):187–189.

McElmurray, Beverly J. and Donna S. Huddleston
  1991 Self-Care and Menopause: Critical Review of the Research. *Health Care for Women International* 12(1):15–26.

Mittness, Linda
  1983 Historical Changes in Public Information About the Menopause. *Urban Anthropology* 12(2):161–179.

Penrose, Charles B.
  1900 [1897] *The Textbook of Diseases of Women*. Philadelphia: W. B. Saunders.

Reynolds, Holly Baker
  1987 *To Keep the Tali Strong, Women's Ritual in Tamilnad, India*. Unpublished Ph.D. dissertation, University of Wisconsin.

Rosenberger, Nancy
  1986 Menopause as a Symbol of Anomaly: The Case of Japanese Women. *Health Care for Women International* 7(1–2):15–24.

Severne, Lisbeth
  1982 Psychosocial Aspects of the Menopause. In *Changing Perspectives on Menopause*, Ann Voda, Myra Dinnerstein and Sheryl O'Donnell, eds. Austin: University of Texas Press.

Shostak, Marjorie
1981 *Nisa, the Life and Words of a !Kung Woman.* Cambridge: Harvard University Press.

Sinclair, Karen P.
1985 Maori Women at Midlife. In *In Her Prime: A New View of Middle-Aged Women,* Judith Brown and Virginia Kerns, eds. South Hadley: Bergin and Garvey Publishers.

Skultans, Vieda
1970 The Symbolic Significance of Menstruation and Menopause. *Man* 5(4):639–651.

Smith, Linda
1987 *Biological and Cultural Effects of Obesity on Women During Menopause.* Unpublished Ph.D. dissertation, Wayne State University.

Spitzer, Denise L.
1994 *Menopause: Biology, Culture and the Individual.* Edmonton: The Centre for the Cross-Cultural Study of Health and Healing, University of Alberta.

Suggs, David
1986 *Climacteric Among the "New" Women of Mochudi, Botswana.* Unpublished Ph.D. dissertation, University of Florida.

Upjohn Company of Canada
n.d. *Menopause and Hormone Replacement Therapy: The Facts.*

Vatuk, Sylvia
1975 The Aging Woman in India: Self Perceptions and Changing Roles: In *Women in Contemporary India,* Alfred de Souza, ed. New Delhi: Indian Social Institute.

Wilbush, Joel
1980 *The Female Climacteric.* Unpublished Ph.D. dissertation. Oxford University.

Wright, Ann L.
1982 An Ethnography of the Navajo Reproductive Cycle. *American Indian Quarterly* 6(1–2):52–70.

World Health Organization
1981 Research on Menopause: Report of a WHO Scientific Group. *Technical Report Series #670.* Geneva: World Health Organization.

IONE

A Winter Retreat

☒

I am awakened early in the morning by a loud thumping sound on the roof, accompanied by raucous, piercing cries. Startled, I run out from the bedroom in my woolen nightgown. There is ice on the railing outside of the wide sliding glass doors that take up most of that side of the house. From here I can see a blanket of snow extending over the backyard toward the beach and the freezing bay. As I slide the glass back, the bitter cold sea wind sparkles against my face. A few feet above my head there is a flapping of huge gray-white wings—a flock of gulls, usually more circumspect, is swarming on top of my cottage. Bold and full of themselves, some clatter down to the railing as I duck inside, while others scramble noisily on the roof before taking off, looking for whatever sparse food the winter might offer them.

This is Sag Harbor in the winter of 1984, and I am far away from the ordinary circumstances of my life. A few hours from my three children—pre-teen and teenaged boys who are with their father in my New York City loft—farther from my grandmother in Saratoga Springs, NY, and farther still from my mother, who is in sunny Mexico. An inexpensive rental, a winter retreat. I have come here to write. I miss everyone.

After ten years of struggle, raising babies, divorcing, making a living as a freelance writer, seeking agents and publishers, I have received a contract for the book of my life—literally, a memoir, inspired by my great grandmother's 1868 diary—that traces the lives of the women in my family back four and more generations. My sojourn in Sag Harbor is supposed to be that legendary retreat spoken of, written of, by other women writers—the time away to do what I have been longing to do: what the world of ex-husbands, lovers and children, the world of bills and everyday details and the need to make a living has impeded—what now, a contract says, I have to do.

But the universe has other plans. Reluctantly, I am forced to turn my attention to my body's changes and the sea of emotions that accompanies them. This blood that I wished upon myself at the age of eleven is fading from me. My body feels as it has never felt before. How to describe it? Something crucial is separating from me, something that once moved forward is grinding to a halt. How different from the powerful feeling of *flowering* when I first began it.

"Congratulations," said Pop, my stepfather, as I lay quietly in the darkened room, "You're a woman now."

"Yes, that certainly is blood," my mother had confirmed earlier in the day. It was everything I ever wanted, the greatest gift of all—it was the perfumes of my mother's smoky mirror dresser, the Shalimar, the Prince Machiabelli, it was the furs and high heels of her locked closet, the swift and purposeful sound of my grandmother's footsteps as we walked downtown in Saratoga (she knew where we were going). It was the rake of her stylish hats at the racetrack, the light and buttery biscuits that emerged from her heated kitchen. The muted cramps I felt seemed to intimate all the stirrings of love and sex to come. Not yet the paroxysms of pain that will soon send me to the nurse's office at school, they nonetheless hinted of danger. I thought myself on the verge of the dangerous sensuality I surmised filled *real* women's lives. I was joining the ranks of the most fascinating women in the world.

Sag Harbor is calm and quiet, but alarms are going off inside me. Each day after a morning bout of unsatisfactory writing on a huge IBM Selectric typewriter, I walk the uneventful road to town—my sole destination, a tiny health food store. Sugar-free cookies, exotic vitamins, split pea soup.

Once or twice a day, I go out for a drive in Greenie, a 1969 Buick made in the same year my eldest son, Alessandro, was born. She was purchased for $300 from an African American mechanic in Sag Harbor, a man I think of as a kind of guardian angel just because he is there—one of the few dark faces in the very white town.

Greenie and I have developed a routine, heading out to the cold and windblown ocean beaches, breathing in the gray of saltbox houses, imagining the evolved, often literary lives inside (for many writers live out here), glinting at the piercing blue of the sky and the battering froth of the waves, surveying the diminishing sand dunes. Sag Harbor has not escaped the sadness of resort towns in winter, and I am grieving. If this period, this bleeding has been my passport to womanhood, then what uncharted territory am I entering now?

Memories of other alone times surface between pages as I lie in bed at night reading, the electric blanket on high, my liberated city cat snuggling under the covers at my feet for warmth. (Later in the night, wrenching upward from deep sleep, I will throw the covers back from my sweat drenched body.) More than once, I have pulled away from those I love, when what I think I *really* wanted—certainly what I *needed*—was to get closer.

There was the time after my confirmation into the African Methodist Episcopal church in Harlem—me dressed in white, pulling away from my mother's congratulatory hug without explanation. I had been upset by the visiting white bishop, whose manner I perceived as condescending to the black congregation. The disappointment and hurt was so deep that I couldn't even speak of it.

And there was my high-school graduation—"No one needs to come," I'd told them, "I don't want to hang around taking pictures outside afterward with all the others." I thought it was corny. Then walking alone down the steps from Music and Art after passing the groups of graduates and parents, wishing they hadn't taken me at my word, that someone had come anyway. Learning only afterward that my grandfather had attended, but left without waiting for me.

And now, during this wintry rite of passage, my attempts to communicate still fall short. A writer who is still at the beginning of the process of unraveling her tongue, finding her truest voice, I am unable to speak of my change of life to my mother, my grandmother—and neither has offered a hint of her own experience of this passage. I search my memory for any mention and find a hot Saratoga summer afternoon when I am somewhere between eight and ten years old, lingering in the hallway as usual, a few feet away from the front porch where my grandmother and two of her friends sit rocking and talking and drinking beer. My grandmother is peeling something, or shucking corn for dinner that night, busy even in this moment of leisure.

"I didn't know what to think when it first stopped," one ample bodied woman says, her voice filled with amusement and another tone I have come to recognize as having to do with sex.

"At first I thought I was *pregnant!*" she exclaims. "You know how Jim is!" Another woman agrees. "Yes, girl, I know what you mean—" There are laughs and chuckles, and they are about to go on when my grandmother, sensing my presence, turns and catches sight of me. With a look and a small shake of her head, she hushes the other women. Cardboard fans flutter, chairs scrape the summer rug as they are adjusted. Beer gurgles into glasses and rises to lips, is swallowed as the women look at me, their faces brimming with secrets. A few moments later, I am outside on the sidewalk passionately bouncing my golf ball and storing the precious pieces of odd information.

They have been waiting until Sag Harbor to be retrieved.

Other messages rise from the depths of my psyche. Despite their natural secretiveness, the women in my family have imparted a few important messages to me. I have revered some of them as if they were encoded clues about womanhood itself.

"A woman never tells her age. Be vague about dates," and, "Always put cold cream on your face at night."

Although I have disobeyed my foremothers in so many other ways, these familiar instructions have held me captive. But now my writing requires me to break the age spell. Can I really tell how old everyone is? Is there any way to write about history without doing so? And these days, cold cream aggravates my normally smooth skin, which has begun to break out as it did when I was entering puberty. The giant jar of Ponds, a staple until now, stands untouched beside the box of tissues on my night table. This is a calamity. Everything is changing. Surely I am betraying my mother and my grandmother by going through something so unglamorous as menopause.

A week or so later, my mother returns from Mexico and I invite her out to my alone place by the water. This is risky, I know. Our pattern through the years has been rounds of fierce fights and tenuous reconciliations. I still do not understand how and why we are so different from each other. I have hopes of a softening of the latest freeze. I want to show off and, yes, to share this symbol of my success with her.

But as my mother steps down from the bus I can tell from the expression on her face that everything has already gone wrong. She is tired and cranky. Later at the house, nothing about me or my place of retreat seems to please her. Everything has a hollow look and feel to it. What had I been expecting? We don't know how to talk to each other any better here than anywhere else. When I put her back on the bus the next day we are both grateful for the end of the visit. Of course I have made no mention of my body's changes.

On another day my grandmother agrees over the phone to come out to the house. Be-Be, in her nineties and a veteran horseplayer, proclaims that she is "weakening in the stretch"— her great strength, which has seemed limitless for all my life, is failing. How I hate that word. I push it from the edges of my thoughts—my own fear of failing at my writing, my fear of her mortality and now, astonishingly, my own.

I pick my grandmother up from my father's apartment in New York and we take the long drive out to the island. Greenie, rattling and shaking on the Long Island Expressway, makes the trip valiantly. Be-Be, never one for mincing words, manages nonetheless not to complain about the discomfort of the drive. Excited to have her with me at the house, I leave the car in the driveway and rush to open the front door. I turn to come back for her to see that she's gotten out on her own and, horribly, as if it were slow motion film footage, she is falling, falling, and I am running, running to get to her, trying to make it in time—not making it.

Once inside I tend to her by putting cool compresses on her bruised and swollen face. A day or two and it starts looking, feeling better—I tend her with the soothing Mentholatum she rubbed on me as a child. One morning, she loosens her diamond ring on her finger, thrusts it toward me. "I want you to have this now."

Be-Be's ring. There is joy to have it and just below the surface—rumbling—a deep pain. Be-Be knows she will not live many more years. She wants to give this to me while she herself can hand it to me.

Cooking against mortality, I make baked chicken, roasted potatoes, asparagus—one day I find a special fish, the catch of the day. On another day I carefully prepare delectable broiled oysters on toast. Be-Be agrees that the view of the bay is beautiful. But one afternoon, she awakens from a nap and suddenly declares that she would like to go back to New York City. There is no questioning her. I prepare our bags and we leave the following morning.

A few days later, back on the island, I am alone again, feeling somewhat more at peace with myself and my winter retreat. I am taking the place over, making it my own. My journals and typewriter are nearby, research books and papers are jumbled all over the small living room. As I watch the glistening water of the bay over a cup of the new decaffeinated coffee, I am no longer thinking of visitors. I remember Cecilia, the nutritionist I consulted before coming out to the island. I am doing as she told me— drinking eight glasses of spring water a day, curtailing sugar and alcohol. I realize that Cecilia's instructions have replaced those of the women in my family about dates and age and cold cream.

Sitting at the table, eating a simple soft boiled egg with grainy whole wheat bread, I dip my spoon in and I see Cecilia soft inside her crisp white coat as she affirms matter of factly, "Yes, this is what is happening, your periods are getting lighter." A slight pause, her dark eyes crinkle, "And then one day they'll be gone." Cecilia gives me a bright, friendly smile, so open and natural that I am jolted as it meets my silent panic head on.

Why is this woman smiling?

I twist Be-Be's ring on my finger. Take in a deep breath. These diamonds, she has told me, given to her by my grandfather, used to belong to his mother, my great grandmother. I try to let my consciousness slip down into their shining facets. Diamonds are said to retain the essence of those who wear them. Somewhere in these facets I sense that the task before me will take several more years of writing and researching. More years of finding the courage to be the woman I am becoming.

All of this is deeply connected to the mystery of Cecilia's smile. I wonder, What does Cecilia know that I don't know?

MARGARET GIBSON

To the Body, at Menopause

❖

1.

I was born in you,
not simply
(as the certificate says)
in Philadelphia,
city of the cracked bell.
First breath, and you
were tolling in surprise
that we were here,
mind and body
held by a spliced
chord of breath,
together and alone.

2.

Swung in the air,
then swaddled,
you were intimate abode
and lodging, an inn
as the troops left for war,
their sundered wives
left to dandle
their babies and breast feed,

to talk in hushed
tones and lullabies, and to grieve.

Held close, I could not tell
my mother's heartbeat
from yours—same syllables.
Even apart, I could hear
the air raid warning
of her nerves. I heard
her spoken words
as she must have heard
the loud tally
of the rumored dead.
Body was number, body
was final sum, bone
and emptiness on foreign soil.
Held close, I began to
be afraid.

3.

I learned to think of you
as seedbed, cradle of stars,
a nest—and I a nurse
who could swallow
the night sky of fearsome
immensities
obedient to unfamiliar laws.

You are so dark, my mother said.
In time, I let
her words flush out
with your month blood.
I let her words
fade into the ardent
dawn of our own cries
kindled in the uprush
and lambent wash of pleasure
as I swung with the tolling

bellropes of the blood,
body (and now I called you
mine) close as a lover.

4.

So many lovers, then one
beloved. So many
missed opportunities
to root a child in you.
Whatever I tell you now
will be too simple.
I had step-children and
so many promises to keep
(I said), I wouldn't
believe my pain. Now even
when you sent it
throbbing monthly through,
as one knocks and knocks
at a door held
firmly shut.

5.

Speech and thought are also
body and abode,
so I held you in my mind,
a tune devised by Plato
and the Gnostics,
then by Aristotle filed
in the helical shelving
of your library,
encoded in the bound
book of the genes.
In words you would grow to
own completion, final
form. I did not remember

that poems are rarely finished
or perfected. I did not
remember that body
is time and history.
Whether it was
an imperishable hush
you carried
or the music of the spheres,
I wanted to make
you immortal.

6.

Then my month blood sputtered,
stalled, stopped for good

and I knew I was mortal. Mortal.

7.

Oh, but science offers
fresh possibilities
chemical formulas, hormones,
lubricants, advice.
Time for a tune-up? There are
engineers. For a make over?
Cosmetics, suction,
and (if necessary) sharp
knives that can make straight
the seams, tucking in
flaccid folds.
And now there are complex
cameras that can show
what you have been making
inside your underworld of
swamp and darkness.
I see the mottled shadows,

and I must claim them,
however otherworldly
they appear. The doctor
calls them my breasts.
I want them touched, as I
touch them now. With respect.

8.

As if you have swallowed the sun,
you have your own
better way of waking me to change.
Thermonuclear surges, tropical
sweats and hours at night
when the ceiling and the walls
dissolve, and we are
eye to eye with the stars.
They wink. They are
mortal, too.

9.

Making love with him,
beloved one, I am
also loving you, not just
the lush flare of flesh
that ripens with
the open vowels of pleasure
so like pain, but also
the toothy consonants,
the knock of bone on bone,
the obstacles to union
that remind me
how like unfaithfulness
separation is.

10.

You are not, as I have
sometimes said,
a nest. Nor war zone.
Neither machine
nor garden. You are
not my better
half, nor worse,
nor are you the house
of pleasure or of pain.
These pass, and you are
not an ocean shell
I can display on a sill,
not a book I can
copyright or own.
In the dream of my anger
at your stubborn
going toward entropy
and decay,
you are simply empty—
a flowerpot made of clay,
no soil inside, no root
nor stem, no blossom,
and no stone to
stop the seep of water.
You are flared open at the rim,
and in the base there is
an open hole
through which light
comes and goes, and wind.

And wind wakes me
to a morning
surrounded by sun,
to a green translucence
of wind and leaves.
I bow to the dream
and to the bloodroot sun
now unfolding

its damp petals,
lifting on a thin stem
into the rimless blue
and clouds of unbounded
blossom—I bow
to water's way of rising
without holding on,
to water's way
of falling as rain
into the whole of the wet
earth and emptiness we are.

GLORIA STEINEM

Age — and a Blessing

❖

"We grow neither better nor worse as we get
old, but more like ourselves."
Mary Lamberton Becker

Dorothy Dinnerstein, the sociologist and author of *The Mermaid and the Minotaur,* once said that growing up in a family teaches us two crucial things: how to get along with and love people who don't share our interests, and what to expect from the various stages of life.

I was struck by the wisdom of the first part of her remark and bored by the second. Didn't everyone know about "the stages of life"?

Well, everything sounds trite before we're ready for it. Almost two decades later, I realized I didn't understand the process of aging at all. Thanks to my very small family, the patterns of my parents' lives, and the fact that I've worked mostly in movements where age differences melt in a furnace of shared interests, I had never thought about or lived with the surprising, upsetting, implacable, and irrevocable mystery of aging. Instead, I had been behaving as if the long plateau of an activist middle of life went on forever.

Though my circumstances set me apart from many of my friends—for instance, I hadn't chosen to have children and so didn't have their growth as a measure of time—I discovered that few people I knew had a vision of anything but a cliff at the end of this plateau. The rarity of extended families, the lack of multigenerational communities, and too few media images that extend beyond forty or fifty—all these things had stopped our imaginations. Meanwhile, my apparent belief that I was immortal, with all the time in the world, was causing me to plan poorly— to put it mildly.

145

Fortunately, our bodies are great teachers: even their smallest inti-mations of mortality are shocks we never forget. I remember having my hair washed at a shop in another city, apologizing as usual for having long hair that is time-consuming to dry, and being told cheerfully, "That's okay—it's rather thin." Then there was the moment when I realized I could only count on going sleepless for one night—not two—when I needed to meet a deadline. And my always nearsighted eyes began to get farsighted at the same time. "I always thought my patients were exagger-ating," the optician said when I asked him if I was going blind or just aging, "until I passed forty—now I know exactly what you mean."

These bodily signals sent me into the first stage of dealing with aging: denial. I was going to continue living *exactly as I always had*—and make a virtue of it. If age were ever to interrupt sexual life, for instance, I would just continue it in a different way. After all, the world could use a pio-neer dirty old lady. Dorothy Pitman Hughes and I began fantasizing a future as bawdy old women sitting on bar stools in skirts that were too tight, sending out for an occasional young sailor. (Of course, neither one of us drank, or felt attracted to members of the opposite sex who hadn't lived through at least some of the same history—but the fact that dirty old men were almost our only role models was a measure of how finite we felt our options to be.) If I ever grew too infirm to work and my delu-sions of perpetual youth had still prevented me from saving any money, then I would just become a bag lady. It was a life like any other, and I could always help organize the other bag ladies.

Gradually, the first stage of denial blended into a second, more ener-gized one: defiance. Two of my role models for this future were George Burns, who had just signed a contract to play the Palladium in London on his hundredth birthday (he was well into his eighties at the time, a bravado which made me overlook his not-so-great sex jokes about young women), and Ruth Gordon, who wore miniskirts in her eighties, had a younger husband (playwright Garson Kanin), and acted up a storm in movies (remember *Harold and Maude?*). She also said satisfying things like "I think there is one smashing rule: Never face the facts."

In this spirit, I celebrated my fiftieth birthday in a very public way by turning it into a feminist benefit (which I hope my funeral will also be), and tried to offer some encouragement to other women facing the double standard of aging by getting as far out of the age closet as possi-ble. Of course, I continued to hear "fifty" as old when applied to other people and had consciously and constantly to revise my own assump-tions. Though I began making an effort to use time better and to understand that my life wasn't going to go on forever—that is, to use turning fifty to good purposes—my heart wasn't in it. In fact, I didn't revise one single thing about my living habits: no exercise except running through airports; no change in my sugar-addicted eating habits; no admission that this long plateau in the middle of my life might be leading into a new terrain. In a way, I felt I *couldn't* acknowledge limitations or any of the weaknesses to which the flesh is heir; the everyday emergencies of a magazine and a movement were all-consuming, and I didn't think I could stop swimming in midstream. But to a larger degree, I just didn't know how. I didn't have a model of how to get from here to there; from where I was to seventy, eighty, and hopefully beyond. I needed a model not of *being old*, but of *aging*.

Thanks to good genes, I got away with all this defiance for quite a while—which may be exactly why I needed the word *cancer* to come into my life. Nothing less than such a bodily warning would have made me think about the way I was living. Sleeplessness and endless stress, a quart of ice cream at a time, and my lifetime rule of no exercise: I was so unaccustomed to listening to any kind of messages from within that I'd ceased to be able to hear even a whisper from that internal voice that must ultimately be our guide. In fact, I had no patience at all with anyone who suggested it was there to be listened to.

Cancer changed that. It gave me a much-needed warning, and it taught me something else: it was not death I had been defying. On the contrary, when I got this totally unexpected diagnosis, my first thought was a bemused, "So this is how it's all going to end." My second was, "I've had a wonderful life." Such acceptance may sound odd, but I felt those words in every last cell of my being. It was a moment I won't forget.

Eventually, that diagnosis and my reaction to it made me realize that I'd been worrying about aging; that my denial and defiance were related to giving up a way of being, not ceasing to be. Though I would have decried all the actresses, athletes, and other worshipers of youth who were able to imagine a changed future—a few of whom have even chosen death *over* aging—I had been falling into the same trap.

For this health warning—plus the dawning of an understanding that to fear aging is really to fear a new stage of life—I was fortunate to pay only a small price. Thanks to the impact of the women's health movement on at least some of the health-care system, my treatment consisted of a Novocain shot and a biopsy at a women's clinic, while I watched an infinitesimal lump being removed in what turned out to be its entirety—rather like taking out an oddly placed splinter. Since the mammogram had shown nothing—15 percent show false negatives, which is another reason for self-examination—the diagnosis of malignancy was a shock. But what came after was not nearly as difficult as what many women have faced. First, there was a lymph-node sampling that did require going into the hospital, but didn't interfere with going dancing the evening I got out. Since the sampling was negative, the rest of the treatment consisted of six weeks of lying like the Bride of Frankenstein on a metal slab each morning while I got radiation treatments. My self-treatment was much more drastic: doing away with all animal fat in my diet, and getting less stress and more sleep. All this has helped me remain cancer-free for the last five years.

Nonetheless, I was frightened enough by this timely warning to start doing what I needed to do, indeed what I should have been doing all along: listening to what my physical self had to say. Perhaps one of the rewards of aging is a less forgiving body that transmits its warnings faster—not as betrayal, but as wisdom. Cancer makes one listen more carefully, too. I began to seek out a healthier routine, a little introspection, and the time to do my own writing, all of which are reflected in these pages.

Now, I've come to believe that bodies know whether their times of transition are leading to something positive or negative. If I tell you that menopause turned out to be mainly the loss of a familiar marker of time, plus the discomfort of a few flushes and flashes—and that to me, the ease of this transition seems related to the much-longed-for era of relative peace and self-expression it ushered in—you may think I've gone off my rocker. But consider the results of a 150-nation menopause study: negative symptoms *increased* when women went from more to less social mobility and power, but *decreased* when women's power and freedom grew. In the United States, where women are valued for youthfulness, for instance, there were many negative menopausal symptoms, but in countries like Pakistan, where women are restricted during childbearing years but allowed more authority and social mobility after menopause, women had very few. Within this country, African-American women reported the fewest negative symptoms and Jewish women reported the most; arguably because of the relative importance of the role that older women play in those communities.

In fact, when a medical anthropologist named Yewoubdar Beyenne came here from Ethiopia, she was so surprised by all the negative attributes of menopause that she did a study of its impact in a wide variety of countries and concluded that it is a "biocultural phenomenon." As she put it, "Coming from a non-Western background, I was not aware that menopause causes depression or any other emotional or physical illness. I only knew that menopause was a time when women in my culture felt free from menstrual taboos." From Mayan women in Mexico to blue-collar and professional women in Britain and Hawaii—all of whom had lives to look forward to that were active and free compared with their own premenopausal pasts—the crucial question was: What kind of era is menopause ringing in?

I'm fortunate to have a future of active work I love and look forward to, but the most crucial element in all these studies seems to be an increase in self-expression and freedom, whether it's part of our work or not. Once again, it's the importance of moving closer to the true self, regardless of our age. When male and female college students were asked to write for just twenty minutes a day, for each of four days, about a traumatic personal experience, for instance, the result was everything from a better emotional state to a strengthened immune system. When the same test was repeated with instructions to write only about trivial events, there was no change in mood or immune response at all. The result is not so different from the Pakistani women in that 150-nation menopause study who could finally get out of isolation and into conversation in the marketplace.

For me thus far, the only disappointment with this new country called aging is that it hasn't liberated me from that epithet of "the pretty one"—though in the past, I sometimes pleasurably fantasized about getting old to get rid of it. If that sounds odd, think about working as hard as you can, and then discovering that whatever you accomplish is attributed to your looks. The up-side has been a better understanding of women who really are great beauties—not just feminists who don't fit a media stereotype—and who are treated without reference to their inner reality, as well as denied sympathy. Perhaps a more personal up-side is seeing age as freedom.

In my current stage of aging and listening, I've learned the importance of starting with the body and all its senses. Which is why I go to my body to ask what this new country of aging will be like.

I look at my hands of which I am so proud, for instance, and seeing their backs sprinkled with small brown age spots is shocking at first. So I ask them what they have to say for themselves. "A banner held in liver-spotted hands," they reply. I get a title for a future article, plus my first inkling that liver spots have a sense of humor.

I notice that the hormonal changes of menopause seem to have freed a part of my brain once preoccupied with sex—thus bringing a more relaxed, I-enjoy-it-when-it-happens-but-don't-obsess-about-it attitude —so I ask these brain cells what they're planning to do with the extra time. "Celebrate not being stuck with bras and sailors," they say. Suddenly, I feel liberated.

I wonder if I should let the bleached streaks in my hair grow out after all these years. I don't want to put a "ceiling on my brain," as Alice Walker would say. Then the phrase "punk-rock purple" comes out of nowhere. Maybe even aging hair doesn't have to be serious.

Looking in the mirror, I see the lines between nose and mouth that now remain, even without a smile, and I am reminded of a chipmunk storing nuts for the winter. This is the updated version of my plump-faced child. When I ask what they have to say for themselves, nothing comes back. They know I don't like them, so until I stop with the chipmunk imagery and learn to value them as the result of many smiles, they're not communicating. I'll have to work on this—and many other adjustments of aging still to come.

But I have a new role model for this adventurous new country I'm now entering. She is a very old, smiling, wrinkled, rosy, beautiful woman, standing in the morning light of a park in Beijing. Her snow-white hair is just visible under a jaunty lavender babushka. Jan Phillips, who took her photograph, says she was belting out a Chinese opera to the sky, stopped for a moment to smile at the camera, and then went on singing. Now, she smiles at me every morning from my mantel.

I love this woman. I like to think that, walking on the path ahead of me, she looks a lot like my future self.

SUE WALKER

Wake Up Call

෴

I am a postmenopausal woman. I am a poet and professor. A writer. A mother. A wife. A person who likes to walk her Labrador retriever but who exercises less than she should and who has no membership in any fitness center. I am fifty years old and wondering how the first sentence in this paragraph and the last relate to the other signifiers of who and what I am.

I say that I am a poet and writer, but this is the first time I have written about menopause. I am a reader, but I don't know of a novel in which the theme *menopause* figures prominently. *The Bridges of Madison County* comes to mind as fiction that deals with mature love, but I don't remember a scene in which the heroine discusses menopause with the man she loves. Imagine this: a restaurant that extends over the ocean. It is evening; the last remnants of sun finger the water like a caress. Silver fish somersault beside the deck where the man who is the passionate other in my life and I dine. He lights the candle on the table. We order oysters Rockefeller, oysters bienville, oysters stewed and nude, and drink a bottle of Montrachet wine. "A few years ago," he says, "this bottle would have been worth a lot more. Let's just say it's special." We sit across from each other. I smile, lean over, and run my fingers down the side of his cheek. "I put new silk sheets on the bed," I tell him. "Gold ones—like the sunset; I sprayed them with *Cayman Memories* real island perfume." His eyes show he's reacting to what I say. He fills my glass with wine. We toast. It goes like this. Me: "For a night of lurid postmenopausal love." Him: "You're the damn most exciting postmenopausal woman in the world."

"Cut," the director shouts. "Delete," the computer bleeps. And I say to myself, "Hey, woman, you ain't real! Who do you know that toasts menopause in a restaurant over the ocean while eating oysters? Get away with ya."

Well, it's like I say. I'm a writer and a poet, but what do you expect? I told you I've never written about menopause before. I'm a professor, too, but until this spring in a new course called Aging and Literature, I had never mentioned menopause in class. Not until we read and began discussing Ursula K. Le Guin's "The Space Crone." She begins it with this line: "This menopause is probably the least glamorous topic imaginable; and this is interesting, because it is one of the very few topics to which cling some shreds and remnants of taboo." I feel like I have peanut butter stuck to the roof of my mouth. I don't feel comfortable talking about what is euphemistically called the "change of life," but I push on. I read the lines: "Loss of fertility does not mean loss of desire and fulfillment. But it does entail a change, a change involving matters even more important—if I may venture a heresy—than sex." I wait for a reaction. I think my hands begin to sweat. The women in the class look at the men, then look around—out the window, toward the hall; they seem as uncomfortable as I. A man in the class breaks the silence. He declares he's fifty-five, laughs, and swears that he has gone through menopause. "I'm serious," he says. "I even went to the doctor. I had these sweats—like hot flashes. I thought I would die." Everyone laughs. Another male—late thirties—joins in. He likes Le Guin's essay, begins to talk about men's fears about crones. The next week we move on to other stories and poems about aging that are unrelated to menopause, but Mark brings a newspaper clipping from the *Atlanta Journal* to class. The headline reads: "Ads are aiming at baby boomers' fears of menopause." "Forty million baby boomers will hit menopause in the next ten years," the article says. It mentions Premarin ads, the Estraderm patch, Tums 500 calcium supplement, and Rejuvex, a product for estrogen-wary women. I thank Mark for the article, fold it up, and put it in my book. I sense his eagerness to pursue the topic of menopause and wonder if my reluctance to go back to it has more to do with my own avoidance than the fact that we have a lot of material to cover, and menopause is not on the syllabus for this particular class. Clearly the men in the seminar are more vocal and express more interest in the subject than the women, who outnumber them thirteen to three.

I am a mother who has never discussed menopause with her children—three sons, ages twenty-nine and eighteen (two are twins). Somehow this seems and does not seem unusual to me. My mother never discussed menopause with me, though she did mention hot flashes and make a display of fanning herself from time to time. But what I remember most poignantly about my mother and aging is a song she used to sing. I was probably fifteen at the time. Mom would sit at the piano, play and croon: "Darling, I am growing older; silver threads among the gold." I cringed. To this day, I hate the song and wouldn't think of having my kids listen to me wail the words ". . . I am growing older; silver threads . . ." And wailing it seemed. I think I felt guilty, like somehow *age* shouldn't happen to my mom. Not when I was young and edging into beautiful. So I would stare at her to determine how she was faring when she played. I couldn't see any gray hairs. Not ever. At seventy-five, when she died, there was not a silver strand among the brown. At fifty, I don't have gray hair either, and as long as I can heft a bottle of Clairol or Loving Care, I won't. Not that gray hair relates to menopause in any straightforward way, but in my mind, it signifies losing color, growing old. And I don't sing about this to my sons. I tell myself that if I had a daughter, it would be different. I might talk about menopause—even if I refused to sing—but I'm not sure about that. My attitude probably reflects gender biases that have existed for a long long time. Elaine Showalter, in *The Female Malady*, states that during the Victorian period "menopausal women were more harshly discussed, more openly ridiculed, and more punitively treated than any other female group, particularly if they were unmarried. In this age group, expressions of sexual desire were considered ludicrous or tragic, and husbands of menopausal women were advised to withhold the desired 'sexual stimulus.'"

No wonder that my mother and perhaps her mother before her failed to say much about the change of life. The condition was supposed to make women unlovable, moody, crazy, sick. I remember when my mother was scheduled for a hysterectomy. Her doctor told me—seriously—that "every woman ought to have a hysterectomy by the time she is forty." I was twenty-four at the time, and I didn't know enough to question his authority.

A couple of years ago when I visited my gynecologist, he inquired, "Are you on hormones?"

"No," I replied, and added that I wasn't sure I wanted to be.

At this, my doctor stooped over, staggered a few feet and asked, "Do you want to be one of those little old hump-backed ladies on elevators?"

"I won't be," I answered. But I should have leapt up from the examining table, put on my bra, panties, clothes and walked right out. Instead I took HRT for a year, and every day of that year, I felt miserable. Bloated. My breasts were sore. I gained weight. For me, estrogen was not an instant return to youth, and since I had not been bothered by hot flashes and other complaints, the transition to hormones was not a comfortable one. I couldn't remember to take my daily pill, so I never knew if the period I was having was induced by the medication or if I could be dying of cancer. I had read about the risk of endometrial cancer unless oral progesterone was added to the regimen of pills (it creates the unpleasant side effects that resemble PMS), and I questioned whether taking hormones was the best thing for me. I had had a lump removed from my breast the year before, and though it was not malignant, the experience made me think that I probably preferred dying quickly of a heart attack to dying slowly with breast cancer that spread to my lungs, my liver, my brain. Yet my doctor was insistent that I should take hormones—for the rest of my life—so I reluctantly gave in and tried. After a year, I quit the pills. Taking hormones, I think, should be an individual decision based on medical data, on personal as well as family history; not on subtle, if not outright, coercion.

I feel that I can demand more than my mother did when it comes to caring for (indeed loving) my body, and I wish that with the knowledge and experience I have now, I could sit beside her on that piano bench until she finished playing, give her a hug, and ask her to tell me how she feels about growing older. And maybe when this essay is finished, I'll hand it to my sons. It will introduce an aspect of my life that is alien to them as I experience it, and perhaps it will enable them to be more receptive to discussing feminine issues—PMS, pregnancy, menopause—with their future wives.

Getting through any new, strange, or difficult time is easier when it exists in conjunction with doing things we love. Eating a voluptuous veal scallopini or poached salmon with cucumber sauce, reading poetry, travelling to New Orleans, Bon Secour, down the street or across town to a friend's house, not to mention walking a yellow Lab, are little things that add to the quality of my life and make it richer and healthier. Last night, as I read a rough draft of this essay to a younger friend, she asked: "What do you want *now*—at this period in your life?" I replied that I was learning the answer to her question. After thinking about it for twenty-four hours, I think I can say that what I want is the joy that a pause to relish little things brings. I don't have to become a full professor anymore or attend a particular Mardi Gras ball. I am secure about who I am and what I want to do. I can even laugh when I'm having a dinner party and the meringue falls off the baked Alaska and the brioche doesn't rise.

Of all the defining items on my list, I have left *wife* last to write about.

It is who I am after the last of my children goes to college this fall. It is who I am when I finish my classes and leave the office, who I am when I'm not writing a critical article on Marge Piercy's *He, She and It*, when I'm not writing a poem or reading a book. It separates me from being alone and having to do things like take out the garbage. It represents more time than the eighteen years I spent at home with my parents and the happy days of my youth. "So what do you want *now*?" my younger friend insists.

Why isn't that question easy to answer? I think of friends and colleagues. Many have recently divorced. Others would like to, but as one told me at a poetry reading not long ago: "My husband isn't well; I can't divorce a sick husband at this time in my life."

"Surely it's not wild sex?" my young friend goes on. I ponder her question. I think of a recent dream in which I was making passionate love to a man—not my husband. It was a surprising and enjoyable dream, and I woke up puzzled by it. But I didn't mention my dream to my husband, nor did I ask him if he had dreams about having wild sex. Is this why men leave their aging wives for younger models? Is this why more women are having relationships with younger men? Is it that we—both men and women—in our middle years crave lost youth? I think that loss may be a central issue. For women, menopause represents a tangible loss—the cessation of blood and all that means: a figure going to hell, breasts sagging, backaches, the threat of lung disease, heart disease, cancer. We had better make the most of time.

Loss. I think of when I was in graduate school in New Orleans. I was walking down the sidewalk one day, after having taken my car to the shop for repairs, and a carload of guys leaned out the window and whistled. It was not degrading or threatening; it was appreciative. I had on a lavender suede miniskirt and vest, white boots. Yeah, I looked damned good, and I knew it. Size eight. I miss size eight—and more than that, I miss being desired in that safe but sexual kind of way.

Loss? I had another dream not long ago. I dreamed that I was having a baby! In actuality, I think having a baby would be a horror. I look forward to having an empty nest, to being able to go off for a spur-of-the-moment weekend, to not having to fuss about mealtimes and the feeding of ravenous teens. I look forward to not having to worry if my sons are not in and it's one o'clock in the morning, or stew about the neighbors complaining because loud music is blaring at a party in my backyard and they can't sleep. Yet I dreamed about having a baby. I had had an egg implanted and I was telling a group of doctors and nurses that I would be back in ninety days to give birth. This dream startled me too—just as I am surprised when I find myself looking at babies and envying just a bit the young women who are having them. In some ways, I would like to have my just graduated twin sons be age two again, or three. I want to take them to Disney World and watch their faces light up with excitement, see their eyes reflect the thrill of a roller coaster ride. I want to read them bed-time stories—*Goodnight Moon*—over and over again, and even get up at dawn-thirty to watch a Bugs Bunny cartoon. I know now that time passes all too quickly. Eighteen years is really no time at all. Not nearly enough for a family to be together. Yes, I think menopause brings a heightened awareness of loss and of wanting to "do it over," so to speak. Maybe that's what men think when they launch into second marriages and having babies again after the first set of children are grown.

But what do I want when I know that I can't double my age anymore? I think I want to laugh more. With my children. With friends. With the man I love. I want to tell him—my husband—to remember that the girl in the miniskirt still lives in my brain. She wants his appreciation, wants him to want her—with his eyes, with words, even if bodies fail, some-times, to live up to expectations.

It is just 6:00 A.M. as I finish this essay. I see a brooding sky through the magnolia leaves outside my window. We've had more than a week of rain. I guess what I don't want is menopause to seem like a period more gloomy than a month of thunderstorms; I don't want it to be a time of anxiety and depression. I wonder what my husband would do if I were to go in right now and start kissing him passionately. If I were to get some sexy potion and start massaging him awake. What would he tell me, if I told him: "Wake up. I'm a postmenopausal woman—and I want you, want you bad." I shake him hard. "Wake up. Wake up," I say.

LYNNE TAETZSCH

This Time of My Life:
A Menopausal Journal

❖

Waking up drenched in sweat, throwing off the covers, I try to recapture the exact texture of unquiet within me. Fear, anxiety—unattached to cause. It seems to come out of a dream, but not exactly. A fragment.

I think as I write this that I must effect a mature voice, that of the menopausal woman. I enter that stage of life which swallows me up in the pool of All-Women. No longer am I Lynne Taetzsch—the changeable Lynne Taetzsch—changes reflected even in her name. I changed the spelling of Lynne to Lyn when I had my first "how-to" book published seventeen years ago. I reluctantly changed my last name to Stoessel when I married the first time, back to Taetzsch after splitting up, then to Genfan when Herb and I pretended to be married. But I never signed my paintings with any name other than TAETZSCH. This is what friends at Cooper Union art school called me—"Hey, Taetzsch" (pronounced as one syllable to rhyme with the letter *H*). I loved the sound of it and would prefer to be called simply that forever. As if there were a *forever* in all this. We are talking about endings, about the end of a woman's life. The end of my life.

Taetzsch is a name unique to my family. If your name is Taetzsch you are related to me. I loved having this unusual and difficult name with its five consonants in a row t-z-s-c-h as in Nie*tzsch*e. I also appropriated the name for my own art. By signing my paintings simply "Taetzsch," I ensured that any other Taetzsches would need to add at least their initials to distinguish themselves. This didn't concern me because I considered myself the only serious artist in the family.

Now there are lots of little Taetzsches running round—my nephews and nieces and their children, cousins and second cousins. But none of them will love the name Taetzsch the way I have loved it, or have the right to use it the way I have.

Writing this, I burst into tears. This wild love for a name so heart-breaking, so ridiculous.

That's menopause for you.

Menopause: a break in life's rhythms. Time to question, to look. To be reminded one has a body.

Body parts. The vagina no longer plump and pinkly wrinkled, elastic—but tight, constricting, smooth—its mysteries unrevealed. No longer menacing—a menace in its shiny, brittle plastic.

Not as if I looked at it myself. All I have are reports of someone else's observation. The last positive report I had was in 1975. It was following my breakup with Herb. I am insecure and crazy, scared to be on my own after seven years with him, and I get drunk at one of my sister Laura's parties. This getting drunk allows me all the socially unacceptable behavior I crave. And a way to get back at Laura for always getting tired of my company before I am tired of hers. This is the standard format of our relationship.

Naturally with my needs this high and the fact that we live practically next door to each other, Laura has armed herself with strong defenses. Her new best friend is a woman who does nothing but insult me whenever I am in her presence. So at this party of eight to ten people there are mostly Laura's friends, like this woman, except for Raymond, who is an old friend of mine. I am drinking one vodka tonic after another. They are playing Leonard Cohen, Bob Dylan, the Rolling Stones. Moving quickly into the "look at me, I'm crazy" stage, feeling that my life is over, no one will ever love me again, I take off my jeans and underpants and thrust my vagina at people. Squatting, legs apart, I demand that someone look. Everyone retreats from the scene except Raymond, who disinterestedly bends down to get a better view and says to me, "It looks OK."

Now, in writing this, for the first time I understand the significance of my being reassured that my vagina was still beautiful, desirable: *because I had just had a hysterectomy.* The operation was recommended because of severe endometriosis that caused horrible long, bloody, painful periods. The alternative was to get pregnant or take birth control pills again. Because I was a migraine sufferer, the pills were too risky, so the hysterectomy seemed like the best option. They operated for two and a half hours, didn't have time to take out my appendix as they had planned. And they left me one ovary.

After the operation, my doctor suggested hormone therapy. I didn't know why, since I still had one ovary. "Why don't we wait and see," I suggested, "whether I need it?" At the time I didn't really know what *needing* it would mean. I just knew I didn't want to start taking any medication just for the hell of it. I'll take the prescription for pain pills, thank you, but skip the estrogen.

The fact is, I usually avoid doctors altogether. But last summer at the end of my forty-eighth year, when menopause symptoms began—hot flashes, anxiety attacks, the works—I finally made an appointment with a gynecologist who I will call Dr. Jones. It took six months for her to see me. If I had been pregnant, I could have gotten an earlier appointment.

Dr. Jones was recommended to me, and I was happy to have a woman doctor for a change. She was in her forties, raising two young children. I felt a camaraderie of colleagues almost, in the tone of our conversation. She seemed practical, down to earth. Told me I was "healthy as a horse." Then she gave me the confidential scoop—that all women who had reached menopause should be taking estrogen.

"Even my eighty-year-old mother?" I asked.

"Yes," she said. "Estrogen helps prevent heart disease and osteoporosis."

She said a blood test could determine for sure if I was menopausal. But after she examined me and took a pap smear, she said she could tell visually that I was indeed menopausal because the skin of my vagina was no longer deep pink and wrinkled, but light pink and smooth. I cringed. Anyone looking at me could tell?!

It had happened, then. I wasn't simply imagining these symptoms. Just as I had always thought that *I* would never become farsighted in my forties as everyone else did, and then of course *did* become farsighted—so, too, had I become menopausal like every other woman before me. This must mean I would die, too, as they all had before me.

So I filled the prescription Dr. Jones gave me for the "minimum effective dose" of oral Premarin and, like a good girl, started taking it immediately. Maybe it would produce a miracle cure—make me love sex again and pant hungrily after Adrian, hot and juicy, every night. That *would* be a miracle, after ten years of marriage.

Five days later I woke up in one of those irritable, dark, depressing moods that makes your skin crawl to have another human being occupying the same house with you, no less the same room. It was a Saturday, and I couldn't tell Adrian to get out and leave me alone. I could have, but that would have been irrational. I was feeling miserable, but I wasn't irrational. I knew *I was having a bad chemical reaction.*

I thought perhaps it would take my body a few days to adjust to the estrogen, so I continued to take it. But three or four days later, when things had not improved, I called Dr. Jones and told her what was happening to me.

"I'm surprised," she said. "It makes most women feel better, not worse."

"Yeah, well . . . what do you think I should do?"

"Unless you're going to put a bullet into your head, keep taking it."

Click.

In spite of Dr. Jones's heartwarming advice, I stopped taking the estrogen. Four days later I woke up one morning and said, "I'm *me* again." So I guess there are limits—outer limits of the self that we can recognize as a transgression when we cross them. Yet I wonder: If I had not stopped taking the estrogen, would I have eventually come to feel that my depression and irritability were finally *normal*? After a point, can we really remember what it felt like to be that other self?

After some research, I feel even more strongly that I don't want to take any hormones. Why do I have this opposition to medical intervention? Why do I want to say, "Leave me alone! Let me die in peace!"

Pieces. That's what they make you feel. Not whole.

The problem is, everything is statistics. I brought home some books on menopause from the science library. I couldn't understand a lot of the jargon, but I could tell from the charts and graphs that it was all statistics. A thousand women took estrogen after menopause, a thousand women didn't, and this is what happened. Technicians measure things like bone density; look at the rates of cardiovascular disease, breast cancer, levels of good and bad cholesterol. Flipping to another study on the differences between taking oral hormone replacements compared to epidermal (skin patches), I discover that when you take oral hormones, you're likely to have severe peaks and valleys in the effects. The valleys may go below the point where the hormone can be of help. The peaks may cause a variety of damage.

Why didn't Dr. Jones tell me about this? Why was I treated like a statistic?

That seems to be the only way science knows how to treat anyone. Predictive results are not based on individuals, but populations, averages, means. And they only know how to look at the down side. No one asks, "How come this group of heavy smokers did *not* get lung cancer?" Except the tobacco companies, who have a vested interest in *that* group of statistics.

I have never been particularly curious about how my own body works. I like it best when it stays in the background—an unobtrusive transmitter of my mind's desires. The fact is, I have never been on easy terms with my body. The real me is the one looking out of this body into the world. When I see myself in a mirror, I am always startled. It gets scary if I look too long.

My body is deteriorating, dying.

Well, it can go if it wants, but *I'm* staying.

I want to know about the ones who fall outside of the statistics. The ones who don't die when they are supposed to. No, that's not it. No one gets out alive.

I'll be fine if I can stay home with my computer, my books, my painting. When I paint or write, it doesn't matter how old I am. I can be vital, outrageous, angry, playful, sexy. It's when I step out into the world that being a menopausal woman becomes frightening. My own prejudices coming back to haunt me: the older woman—invisible, superfluous, fading, irrelevant.

When I was a young girl, I refused to associate myself with anything female. Of course I had dolls, but I banged their heads against the sidewalk. Feeling trapped by childhood as well as femalehood, I told myself stories to get through the day, adventure stories in which I was the male hero—some variation on the Lone Ranger, Tarzan, or Superman. In my dreams, up until my late teens, I was always male. A boy cousin and I were best friends until puberty, after which we never spoke to each other again. When I saw my brothers' wives—my three sisters-in-law all pregnant at the same time—in their little coffee klatches exchanging symptoms, I promised myself I would never grow up and be one of them. I refused to learn to cook or clean or garden. I was going to do serious work and to have adventures and to be someone in the world.

How can a little old lady *be* someone in the world?

Although I've been menopausal for a year now, there are days when I can't believe this is happening to me. I am the one who is never sick, who doesn't need doctors. The one who looks fifteen years younger than I really am. Thanks to the genes I inherited from my mother, whose skin is still smooth at eighty-three, I have the complexion of a twenty-five-year-old. "Peaches and cream," my friends say, complaining to me about the coarsening of their skin, the incipient wrinkles at eyes and mouth. When I look in the mirror, I wonder if my good luck is true. People say it, but do I believe it? And why do I need to believe it? Why is it always a compliment to be thought younger than you are?

Sitting here at the keyboard, I feel a hot flush creep over my skin . . . drops of sweat accumulating . . . my glasses beginning to slide down my nose. I have an urge to turn on the air-conditioning. But of course I know if I just wait, the hot flash will pass and in a few minutes I'll feel normal again. No, I can't say I know any more what *normal* is. These days it is normal for me to pass continually from hot to cold to hot again; to be struck at odd times of the night with deep feelings of fore-boding, of fear, of undifferentiated anxiety. I crawl into bed eager to embrace the *petit mort*—the bliss of unconsciousness—only to be awak-ened with a start by an unnameable loathing in my gut. It makes me want to wrench free, to turn myself inside out to get away from the horror, the awful, intolerable despair that comes from nowhere, from no cause I can decipher, though I try.

As the revulsion recedes, I go over my day, searching for causes to attach to this effect. I try to remember what it was like before all this started. I think things must have been different once, but I can't really be sure. This is me now—who I am. Who I have always been.

I see my life split into thirds: before pregnancy, after pregnancy, and now—this time of my life. When I was a kid my brothers called me "skinny Linney" and "four sticks sticking out of a bag." I never thought about food, was never hungry, never gained weight. And to get me through a tough project at art school, Benzedrine was great for staying up all night.

At twenty-six I got pregnant with Blixy and everything changed. I would just keep eating at mealtimes until all the food on the table was gone. If I wasn't eating, I wanted to be sleeping, and uppers didn't help.

Blixy is twenty-four years old now, married, thinking about starting her own family. My body is going into a new phase. It's ready for some-thing else.

I told one of my professors the other day (I'm working on a doctoral degree in English) that there were so many things I wanted to read. She said I should concentrate on what I needed professionally right now, not get sidetracked. The professor is a purposeful young woman in her first job out of graduate school.

"You have the rest of your life to read," she said.

"That may be true for *you*," I said, "but *my* life is more than half over."

She seemed startled.

My body is trying to tell me it's time for a change—time to throw off the old skin in order to emerge shiny and sleek—streamlined for the final . . .

I don't know what it is that awaits me, except death. But I do have this longing to cast off excess. My metabolism has changed. I'm getting thinner. I fight it by overeating because I'm scared of what's coming.

Sex no longer interests me. I'd rather write about it than do it. Maybe that's my new obsession—writing about it. I got a rejection slip from a literary journal the other day. It said, "We're frankly tired of all these stories on sex, whether long or short!"

I looked again at the rejected piece. It didn't seem to me to be a sex story, but rather a playful spoof on academic theorizing. Maybe it was the *reader* who was seeing sex in all those inkblots.

Last year when the hot flashes started, I lost my sex drive completely. Actually, it's been a very long time since sex drove me in any compelling sort of way. If memory serves me, the preoccupation with desire only drove me to distraction when sex was *not* readily available. When I can have it any time I want it, the problem reverses. Now the job is to create *desire*, not *opportunity*.

I may as well confess. For me, love and sex don't have much to do with one another. The heart of my marriage, for me, is its ongoing conversation—an examination of the correspondences and disparities of our minds, our language, our march toward death. A recent thrill, for example, was the discovery that Adrian thinks in pictures, not words. He creates three-dimensional scenarios in his mind, concrete visualizations that he then has to translate into abstract concepts in order to communicate. The key to unlocking his mind, I finally learned, was not to ask "What are you thinking?" but "What do you see?" For me, the intimacy between us is in this kind of intercourse, and our waning sex life is irrelevant. Not so for Adrian, however, who sees my desire for twin beds as the disintegration of our love and marriage.

The medical facts are that menopause does not physically affect a woman's sex drive. Sex may be painful because your juices stop flowing, but that problem can be easily solved with Vaseline or creams. Any other difficulties are purely psychological. Feeling like a dried up old prune, for example, is a state of mind, not body.

Of course, when I start investigating what is meant by a "medical fact," I find that it is a case of averages and correspondences, cause and effect. They have found no biological necessity for you to feel less sexy after menopause than before. That is, they can't explain it. Some women report feeling less sexy, others more—often due to the new freedom from childbearing. Headaches, hot flashes, depression, tension, anxiety—there are multitudes of reported *symptoms* of menopause, which vary considerably according to culture. During the nineteenth century, women were thought to go crazy at menopause. Wouldn't you go crazy too if all that blood which used to be released each month were suddenly stoppered up and attacking your brain? "Treatments suggested for the erotic and nervous symptoms of menopause were so unpleasant that one can easily imagine their deterrent effectiveness," says Elaine Showalter in *The Female Malady*. Recommendations included "a course of injections of ice water into the rectum, introduction of ice into the vagina, and leeching of the labia and the cervix" (75).

We've come a long way, baby, from Victorian England, where it was considered ludicrous for a menopausal woman to be interested in sex. In our culture, we impose the opposite demand: she'd *better* want to look young and to feel sexy. She should at least pretend that she's going to live forever. Talking about death makes people nervous. Yet I find myself wanting to find a culture that accepts death, that grants that it is perfectly appropriate to dedicate the last third of your life to cessation, diminishment, putrefaction. What would it mean, actually, to focus on death instead of life? I think of the opening, flowering activity of youth—the need to find community and communion, to merge and procreate. When I was young I endured a tormented frenzy of desire. Time was too slow, and I could never stay in any one place long enough to find out how things would end.

I'm trying to hang around for endings now. I'm actually finishing a Ph.D. this year. That's pretty steady for someone who took twelve years to get a B.A. because she kept quitting schools and changing majors.

My forte is starting over, not finishing.

Every day, as I study for my doctoral exams in English, I think about changing my major focus or writing a dissertation on something other than the one I'm a hundred pages into. I compulsively buy books from other disciplines—philosophy, anthropology, psychology, film studies—just in case I might miss some secret lore. Or more likely, in order to avoid finishing the book I'm supposed to be reading.

I love beginnings. I go at them with the full-tilt energy of a zealot.

Everything is promised in a beginning.

I had my hair cut today at a new hairdresser's. While engaging in the required chitchat, I mentioned that I had a married daughter.

"You're kidding," said the beautician. "You couldn't be that old!"

"Thanks," I said.

Maybe you have to reach your eighties, like my mother, to say what you really think. She sent me a letter on my fiftieth birthday, along with the bread knife that had been in our family for ages. My sister Laura and I had been down to visit her and my father recently and I guess we had a little mock fight over the bread knife, as siblings will do.

My mother said in the letter, "This isn't a birthday gift but we bought ourselves a set of knives and thought you would like to have the old bread knife, as you and Laura threatened to want it when we go. You won't have to wait any more."

Did she really think we were *waiting* to get the bread knife? Waiting for her to *go*?

How cavalierly we treat the other person's *going*. Isn't there something better we can do?

Before I turned fifty this month, I had a premonition that I would wake up that day as Kafka's Gregor Samsa did—a hard-shelled beetle. Stiff, awkward, crablike, I would scuttle through the rest of my life close to the ground—inflexible, unyielding, unresponsive.

Now that I have lived through half a century, I want to stop being a nice person. I am sick of monitoring my behavior so that people will like me.

I hate my friendly smile. It has kept me from acting the part I envisaged for myself at seventeen when I tried out for the seductive villainess in a college play. "No, no," said the director. "With your blond hair and sweet face, you should try out for the heroine." The sweet, dumb, cheerful, good-natured blond, that's me on the outside, but inside it's all dark, dismal despair. I know I'm not a nice person. Why do I have to look and act like one?

Six months later preliminary exams are over and I am ABD (all but dissertation) at last. I can stop studying ten hours a day, seven days a week and get back to all the things I put on hold while I was.

I buy another book on menopause. The description of what happens to your body without estrogen sends me to a new gynecologist, who prescribes a combination of estrogen and testosterone for my "low libido" on a trial-and-error basis. He apologizes for his colleagues, says there is no "average dose" that works for everyone. After a week and a half, I feel no negative side effects, though my libido refuses to budge.

Adrian's shrink asks me how our sex life is coming along. I tell him I don't think the problem has been resolved yet. I take out a two-year subscription to a health newsletter in order to get the free booklet, "Ten Secrets to a Better Sex Life." I add vitamin B-6 to my vitamin E and calcium supplements. I write "niacin" on my shopping list. Why am I doing this? I don't want a better sex life, I just want a good night's sleep.

The day I get the testosterone-estrogen prescription, Adrian and I play tennis and I beat him six-one. Just the thought of getting this male hormone makes me stronger, faster and more aggressive.

Two weeks later I get a call from George Washington University to arrange a job interview for a three-year instructorship. This is incredible after a year of sending out over seventy applications, getting no interviews, watching all my friends fare about as poorly except for one twenty-six-year-old hotshot who gets six interviews and two tenure-track job offers. I was so demoralized, in fact, that I had decided I would probably have to give up the idea of teaching at a university and go back to writing how-to books. With no compulsion to finish my dissertation, I had signed up for a local tennis tournament and had made it to the finals—playing this match the night before we drove to Washington for the interview. Adrian was excitedly coaching me and our adrenaline was up more for this match than for the interview. After a grueling two and a half hours, I lost the match but went home with a second-place trophy.

My interview at George Washington went so well I came out of it telling Adrian I'd be shocked if they didn't offer me a job. Then we celebrated with friends, and the next morning I thought I had a hangover. We were still in DC visiting friends, but I spent the weekend in bed, now convinced it was the flu. I was still taking the hormones and did not connect them with my illness until it lingered after we drove home and ended a few days later in a nightmarish migraine headache so bad I was throwing up all night.

I stopped taking the hormones. I was offered the job.

Now in the excitement of finishing my dissertation, selling the house, looking for a place to live in Washington, the problems of menopause have faded. Yet nagging at me, still, is the specter of death. I promise myself that I will look for a new gynecologist in Washington, do some more research, but my heart isn't in it. I am taking vitamins and supplements out of five different bottles—multivitamins, calcium, bioflavinoids, flaxseed oil, vitamin E—yet I have no confidence in this program. It is what my mother does, and I have always criticized her for it.

"If you eat right, Mom, you don't need all that junk." I tell her she may be doing herself more harm than good, and now I wonder if the headachy feeling I have today is from an overdose of these vitamins. Or is it from an overdose of self-absorption?

As I prepare my course in freshman writing, I try to focus on exactly what it is I must share with these students. I want them to use writing to explore, to test their values and question their assumptions. I want them to dig deep, to make connections between the world outside and the world inside. I want them to feel the excitement of discovery and the anguish of uncertainty. I want them to play with language as well as to work with it.

I want too much.

And then I lose all hope that I could teach anyone anything about writing or meaning or truth. What truth have I found for myself? Hasn't my own search revealed instead the awful complexities, contradictions and ultimate absurdity of life? That all our best and worst inclinations may be due simply to body chemistry? Is there anything positive I can offer these students as I myself lurch back and forth from one state of mind to another?

I try to explain these feelings to Adrian, and he tells me he sees me in water—a swimming pool. "No," he says, "a pool has solid edges. I see you in the ocean, floating, the waves pulling you one way, then another. You're trying to figure out where you are but there is only the sea, no landmarks to guide by."

"Well then," I tell him, "look for another metaphor."

JULIA CONNOR

Coming In

In my imaginary paragraph, no words exist that do not in some
fundamental way forever change your life.
dream voice, September 23, 1987

I arrived just in time for menopause. One day my lover and I were walking down a dirt road at a hot springs about two-thirty in the afternoon
when I realized with a start that I had come into myself. I mean literally,
had come *into* my body. It was a sudden and completely new sense of
equilibrium, a shift of balance in the weights and measures of myself. It
was sheer revelation. I was somehow *changed*. It was hot and we were
walking down this dirt road arguing amicably about something or other
when I suddenly felt the momentous change. It was 1987. I was forty-five.
I remember those large blue dragonflies were everywhere. I thought I
must be crazy. What did I mean *come in?* Where did I think I had been?
But no amount of self-doubt could erase the uncanny sensations I was
having as I put one leg forward, then the other, and felt the weight shift,
the flesh rise and settle across my buttocks, the thigh tighten and release,
the pelvis tilt, the hip pivot, the foot fall. I was monumental. I turned to
my lover and said, *You know, I think I've come into myself.* But I knew the
words didn't do justice to what I was experiencing.

It wasn't so much the annunciation that startled me. My first pregnancy
had announced itself similarly, albeit in the middle of the night, when I
startled my then-almost-husband by sitting bold upright from a dead
sleep and announcing *My God! I'm pregnant!* as if the white dove had
whispered it in my ear. But that made more sense to me. It doesn't seem

strange, not really, to be able to detect the activity of a foreign entity within oneself. And certainly the ruckus that the chromosomes make at the time of conception is something like the arrival of a foreign entity, *cum* entourage.

But I wasn't pregnant now and I knew it—though in many ways I have found pregnancy and menopause akin. For days I walked around inside this bubble. *Did I show?* I imagined I saw people looking at me expectantly. *Could they tell?* I wanted to answer each casual glance with a knowing nod. *Yes,* I wanted each of my nods to say . . . *Yes* . . . *I am.* I was elated to at last be walking around inside my own gravitational force. *Wow,* I wanted to shout, *I'm a realm.* But, of course, I didn't say these things. Instead I became intensely lonely. In our time it is often embarrassing to be happy, especially over something so natural, so silly and intimate, as your own organic change. To the culturally programmed part of me, my discovery seemed preposterous, so except for a very few friends, I kept it to myself.

It was during that same stay at the hot springs, perhaps the following afternoon—in response to something I said about a life in poetry—that my lover turned to me and said, *The truth is imaginative.* It was not a new thought, but it had been offered, had fallen upon us, I felt, like a gift. That's important, I told him and wrote it down in my journal and drew a box around it the way I do with things I want set apart. A few nights later, we'd been reading Dante aloud in bed when I climbed onto him. *Ouch . . . you're heavy!* he said. *I told you,* I said. *I came in.*

MARGE PIERCY

Something to look forward to

⊬

Menopause—word used as an insult:
a menopausal woman, mind or poem
as if not to leak regularly or on the caprice
of the moon, the collision of egg and sperm,
were the curse we first learned to call that blood.

I have twisted myself to praise that bright splash.
When my womb opens its lips on the full
or dark of the moon, that connection
aligns me as it does the sea. I quiver,
a compass needle thrilling with magnetism.

Yet for every celebration there's the time
it starts on a jet with the seatbelt sign on.
Consider the trail of red amoebae
crawling onto hostess' sheets to signal
my body's disregard of calendar, clock.

How often halfway up the side of a mountain,
during a demonstration with the tactical police
force drawn up in tanks between me and a toilet;
during an endless wind machine panel with four males
I the token woman and they with iron bladders,

I have felt that wetness and wanted to strangle
my womb like a mouse. Sometimes it feels cosmic

and sometimes it feels like mud. Yes, I have prayed
to my blood on my knees in toilet stalls
simply to show its rainbow of deliverance.

My friend Penny at twelve, being handed a napkin
the size of an ironing board cover, cried out
Do I have to do this from now till I die?
No, said her mother, it stops in middle age.
Good, said Penny, there's something to look forward to.

Today supine, groaning with demon crab claws
gouging my belly, I tell you I will secretly dance
and pour out a cup of wine on the earth
when time stops that leak permanently;
I will burn my last tampons as votive candles.

Notes on the Contributors

※

BONNIE BRAENDLIN is an associate professor of English at Florida State University, where she teaches American literature and literature written by women. She is writing a book on women's novels written during the 1970s Women's Liberation Movement.

JANET BURROWAY is the author of plays, poetry, children's books, and seven novels including *The Buzzards, Raw Silk, Opening Nights*, and most recently *Cutting Stone*. Her text *Writing Fiction* is used in more than three hundred colleges and universities in the U.S. She is the Robert O. Lawton Distinguished Professor at the Florida State University in Tallahassee.

JULIA CONNOR is the author of four books of poetry. She lives in Sacramento, California, where she teaches writing and painting privately as well as in the state prison system and at a shelter for homeless women.

MARGARET GIBSON is the author of five books of poems, among them *Long Walks in the Afternoon, Memories of the Future*, and *The Vigil*, a finalist for the 1993 National Book Award in poetry. She is a visiting professor at the University of Connecticut. *Earth Elegy: New and Selected Poems* is forthcoming.

ELLEN GILCHRIST is the author of eleven books, including the National Book Award-winning *Victory Over Japan* and, most recently, *Starcarbon* and *The Age of Miracles*. She lives in Fayetteville, Arkansas.

GERMAINE GREER was born in Melbourne, Australia, in 1939, and educated at the universities of Melbourne, Sydney, and Cambridge. Her first book, *The Female Eunuch*, published in 1970, was an international bestseller. Her subsequent books include *The Obstacle Race, Sex and Destiny, The Madwoman's Underclothes*, and *Daddy, We Hardly Knew You*. Currently she is a special lecturer and unofficial fellow at Newnham College, Cambridge University.

CECELIA HOLLAND was born in 1943, graduated from Connecticut College, and has published more than twenty novels, mostly historical fiction. She has three daughters and lives in Northern California, where she teaches and writes. Her latest novel, *Jerusalem*, will be published by Forge in February 1996.

IONE is the author of *Pride of Family: Four Generations of American Women of Color* (Avon Books). She is also the playwright and director of *Njinga the Queen King*, a play with music and pageantry.

MARILYN KRYSL has published two books of stories and five of poetry. Her newest fiction appears in the anthology *Lovers* and the *North American Review*. She teaches at the University of Colorado, Boulder, and volunteers for Peace Brigade International.

MONIFA A. LOVE is McKnight Doctoral Fellow in English at Florida State University. *Provisions*, a volume of her poetry, was published by Lotus Press in 1989. Her work has appeared in *Essence, New Letters, The American Voice, African American Review*, and *Sage: A Scholarly Journal on Black Women*. Her work is included in *Adam of Ife: Black Women in Praise of Black Men* and *In Search of Color Everywhere: A Collection of African American Poetry*. Ms. Love frequently collaborates with her husband, visual artist Ed Love.

NORMA FOX MAZER has published twenty-three novels for young adults, two collections of short stories, and a poetry anthology, as well as numerous articles and short stories appearing in magazines ranging from *Redbook* to *English Journal*. She has received a Newbery Honor Medal, the Edgar Allen Poe Award, the Christopher Award, the Lewis Carroll Shelf Award twice, and has been nominated for the National Book Award. Her books have been translated into German, French, Spanish, Dutch, Danish, Swedish, Norwegian, Finnish, Italian, and Japanese.

SARA McAULAY was born in Washington, D.C., raised in northern Virginia, and spent most of her adult life in the San Francisco Bay Area. She now lives with her partner in Oakland and teaches English and Creative Writing at the California State University at Hayward. She is the author of three novels and a number of short stories and essays. Given a choice, she says she would rather travel than breathe.

FAYE MOSKOWITZ directs the creative writing program at George Washington University. She is author of *A Leak in the Heart, And the Bridge Is Love*, and *Whoever Finds This: I Love You*, and editor of *Her Face in the Mirror: Jewish Women on Mothers and Daughters*.

MARGE PIERCY has published over ten novels, including *Woman on the Edge of Time, Vida, Braided Lives, Gone to Soldiers*, and *He, She and It*. Her collections of poetry include *The Moon Is Always Female; Circles on the Water; Stone, Paper, Knife; My Mother's Body;* and *Available Light*. She has coauthored a play, *The Last White Class*, with her husband, Ira Wood, the novelist and screenwriter, with whom she lives on Cape Cod.

CATHERINE REID's work has appeared in several anthologies (*Reweaving the Web of Life, Rivers Running Free, All the Ways Home*) and in various journals, including *Massachusetts Review, Green Mountain Review, Sinister Wisdom*, and *Sojourner*. She teaches Women's Literature and writing courses at Florida State University.

ELISAVIETTA RITCHIE has published books of poetry and fiction, including *The Arc of the Storm, Raking the Snow*, and *Tightening the Circle Over Eel Country*. Her book *Flying Time: Stories & Half-Stories* includes four PEN Syndicated Fiction winners.

MARY ELSIE ROBERTSON has published five novels, the latest being *What I Have to Tell You* (Penguin 1991), as well as stories in various places including *Ms.* and *Virginia Quarterly*. She has taught in the M.F.A. programs at Syracuse University, the University of Arizona, Wichita State University, and Warren Wilson College. She grew up in Arkansas but lives now in upstate New York.

Denise Spitzer is conducting doctoral research in anthropology at the University of Alberta, Edmonton, Canada, focusing on the experience of menopause among women in Chinese, Chilean, and Somali communities in Canada. Her master's thesis is published by the Centre for the Cross-Cultural Study of Health and Healing under the title *Menopause: Biology, Culture and the Individual*. Denise is active in numerous organizations including the Canadian Council on Multicultural Health and the Intercultural Health Association of Alberta.

Gloria Steinem has been a writer and activist for almost thirty years. Her books include *Outrageous Acts and Everyday Rebellions* and *Marilyn: Norma Jean*. She is the consulting editor of *Ms.* magazine, which she co-founded in 1972. She also helped to found *New York* magazine, where she was the political columnist. She lives in New York City, where her apartment is "a stop on the underground railway" for international feminists.

S. Holly Stocking teaches science writing and essay writing in the School of Journalism at Indiana State University in Bloomington. She is a former staff writer for the Associated Press, the *Los Angeles Times*, and the *Minneapolis Tribune*.

Mary Swander is the author of three books of poetry and two nonfiction collections. Her latest work, *Out of This World*, is a memoir published by Viking in 1995.

Susan Terris lives in San Francisco. Her recent works include *Author! Author!* and *Nell's Quilt* (Farrar, Straus & Giroux), *Killing in the Comfort Zone* (Pudding House Press), and many journal publications. She is currently completing a poetry collection entitled *Wedges of Parallel Time*.

Alma Luz Villanueva is the author of the novels *Naked Ladies* and *The Ultraviolet Sky*, four books of poetry, and *Weeping Woman: La Llorona and Other Stories*. *Planet*, her most recent book of poetry, won the Latin American Writers Institute poetry award in 1994.

Sue Walker is the founding editor of *Negative Capability* and a professor of English at the University of South Alabama. Her critical articles in the field of American literature and her poetry have been widely published.

Acknowledgments

My thanks to Judy Bayliss, list owner of the menopause internet group, where I met wonderful women eager to share their knowledge and stories with each other. Thanks especially to friends Sandy Beck and Eloise Currie for helping me realize how important it is for us to speak to each other about our change of life experiences. Thanks to Patricia Foster for offering her advice, experience and encouragement throughout the development of this project. And most of all, my thanks to the contributors who have shared their lives with honesty and grace in order to make this book possible.

"Mrs. Ramsey, Menopause and Me" by Bonnie Braendlin. Copyright © 1995 by Bonnie Braendlin. Used by permission of the author.

"Changes" by Janet Burroway. Copyright © 1993 by Janet Burroway. Previously published in *Minding the Body*, Doubleday, 1994, and *A Certain Age*, Virago Press, 1994. Reprinted by permission of the author.

"Coming In" by Julia Connor. Copyright © 1995 by Julia Connor. Used by permission of the author.

"To the Body, at Menopause" by Margaret Gibson. Copyright © 1995 by Margaret Gibson. Used by permission of the author.

"The Wine Dark Sea" by Ellen Gilchrist. Copyright © 1995 by Ellen Gilchrist. Used by permission of the author.

Lynne Taetzsch is the author or co-author of nine books. Her essays and stories have appeared in the anthology *Minding the Body, Negative Capability, Atticus Review, Pacific Review, High Plains Literary Review,* and other publications. She holds a Ph.D. in creative writing from Florida State University and currently teaches at Morehead State University and lives in Morehead, Kentucky.